THE SEX POSITIONS *Challenge*

INÈS CHAPMAN

WOPRINTED

Illustrations : Asya Frizen

DISCLAIMER

Author cannot be held responsible for any injuries or breakages that may occur as a result of following the advice in this book. Always check your partner's well-being when trying out new positions.

Have fun!

SPECIAL REQUEST

Dear Customers,

Thank you for your trust.

I publish my books independently. If you like this book, please feel free to leave me a comment on Amazon. I read each of your comments carefully, they are crucial to support my work and allow me to offer you new quality content.

I hope you enjoy this book as much as I enjoyed writing it!

In advance, a big thank you!

Inès Chapman

CONTENTS

BONUS 1

Introduction...2

The Sex Positions Challenge 4

Intimate Exploration...7

    Intimate Communication... 8

    Mood and Setting the Scene.. 10

    The Subtle Art of Caresses 12

    Getting Started 14

The Sex Position Guide 16

    Sensual Warm-Up 16

    Sizzling Adventures... 64

    Enchanting Acrobatics 112

Conclusion...159

BONUS

To help you keep tabs on your progress in this thrilling challenge and enjoy rewards at every successful step, I've put together this **FREE** resource to complement the book.

You can gain instant access to the Challenge Journal and 20 sex coupons by simply clicking the link or scanning the QR code below.

This bonus is absolutely free and comes with no strings attached. You won't need to provide any personal information except for your email address (so I can send it to you).

To claim your bonus, scan the QR code below. :

Introduction

Welcome, dear Love Adventurers! Fasten your belts — or perhaps I should say, unfasten them —and get ready to partake in passionate and sultry moments!

Kamasutra... Does that word ring a bell? Maybe you've whispered it mischievously during a wild evening? Or perhaps you've already tried some of its acrobatic positions, with varying degrees of success? But how much do you truly know about this ancient treasure?

Kamasutra is much more than a mere catalog of lovemaking positions! It encompasses no fewer than seven books, with only one dedicated to erotic postures. This millennia-old text is an intricate roadmap of intimacy and couple's relationships, where each component—whether it's a gentle caress, a passionate kiss, or a bold posture—fits into a seductive dance of desire. Kamasutra is a journey, one that encompasses not only the physical but also the emotional and psychological dimensions of eros.

It's in this spirit, with the desire to help couples break free from monotony, enrich their intimacy, and improve their communication and pleasure, that "The Sex Positions Challenge" was born.

"The Sex Positions Challenge" is a game tailored to guide you toward a more intimate understanding of your own desires and those of your partner. It's an invitation to curiosity, experimentation, and the celebration of all facets of shared pleasure. Here, there's no competition! Each couple progresses at their own pace, always mindful that every challenge comes with its own set of risks. Not all positions are suitable for every adventurer! Some require flexibility, others demand strength. Feel free to adapt the positions to your physical abilities. Gentleness and control will be your allies in sidestepping any risk of injury.

So, are you prepared for the challenge? Take a deep breath and gear up for the most sensual adventure of your life.

Welcome to "The Sex Positions Challenge"!

1
The Sex Positions Challenge

Game Rules

Now, you're at the core of the game now. Get comfortable, kick back, and brace yourselves to dive into a world of uncharted pleasures and sensual discoveries.

But before plunging headfirst into this carnal challenge, take the time to explore "Intimate Exploration," a series of intimate, perhaps even a tad naughty, questions designed to help you uncover and understand your deepest desires and personal limits. Don't miss this rendezvous in the next chapter, where you'll start to unveil your desires and inhibitions.

Now, it's time to unveil the secrets of "The Sex Positions Challenge."

First, you and your partner will need to decide how many positions you want to explore. Take into account your availability, energy, and, of course, your appetite for adventure! Can't make up your minds? Leave it to fate by rolling a die and letting destiny decide for you!

Next up: selecting positions. Flip through the "Position Guide" and pick the ones that tickle your fancy from the three difficulty levels. Or, if you want to add a bit of spice, turn this selection into a game. All you need to do is number 69 small pieces of paper and toss them in a jar. When the urge for a challenge strikes, draw the number of papers corresponding to the positions you wish to try. Each number on the papers corresponds to a position in the guide.

The positions you complete will gradually be removed from the game.

For every mastered position, you'll earn points:

- 5 points for a "Sensual Warm-Up" position,

- 10 points for a "Sizzling Adventures" position,

- 15 points for an "Enchanting Acrobatic" position.

But hold on to your hats, because the adventure can get even spicier with bonus points:

- An additional 5 points if you explore love beyond your comfort zone,

- An extra 5 points for a romantic escapade outside your usual bedtime hours,

- 10 points for a performance worthy of a romantic movie,

- An extra 10 points for using naughty accessories, such as a blindfold, a feather, handcuffs, a costume, or a sex toy,

- 10 points for cunnilingus, fellatio, or sodomy,

- And the grand prize of 20 points if you both reach nirvana simultaneously.

All these points will add up to give you your daily score, proudly recorded in a journal or your **Challenge Journal.** [1]

As your stash of points grows, you'll hit key milestones: 100, 200, 300 points... which you can celebrate with a romantic or sexy experience of your choice (candlelit dinner, lovers' get-away, challenges or naughty games...). Running out of inspiration? Give our **20 surprise coupons** a whirl! [2]

So, the rules of "The Sex Positions Challenge" are as straight-forward as they are thrilling. And when you've completed all the positions and your challenge is done, well, start over and try to improve your score!

---

[1] Free Challenge Journal (BONUS p.1)

[2] Free surprise coupons (BONUS p.1)

2
Intimate Exploration

The sensual quiz

Think you know everything about your partner? Are you sure? This naughty quiz is your VIP ticket for a guided tour of the most secret nooks and crannies of your garden of desires. So, grab a pen and paper or whisper the answers to each other and get ready to reveal yourselves and maybe even... blush!

Life is short; make the most of it, especially under the sheets!

Intimate Communication
Talk to me about love!

Dear passionate explorers, always remember this: each question is an opportunity, an invitation to share, to laugh, and to draw nearer to each other. Dive deep into these questions, be bold, have fun, and, most importantly, let the journey of intimate exploration take you to places you've never dared to venture before.

- If your partner were a treat, what would they be, and why?

- Imagine you have a magical box where you can whisper your secret desires. At what time of day would you hand it to your partner for them to open?

- Your partner surprises you by coming home with a mysterious object meant to spice up your intimacy. What do you secretly hope it is?

- If you had to describe a fantasy to your partner using only movie titles, which ones would you choose?

- How would you like your partner to react if you revealed an unknown aspect of your desires: with words, a gesture, a song, or an impromptu dance?

- If you and your partner were to star in a scene from a romantic movie, where would it be, and what would happen?

- Think of a song that best encapsulates your current feelings about your intimate life. What is it, and why?

- You have the chance to send a letter to your partner from the future. What advice or revelation about your intimacy would you offer?

- Imagine that every touch from your partner leaves a luminescent mark on your body. What pattern or design would you like to see after a night of passion?

- If your sex life were a restaurant menu, would there be dishes you'd hesitate to try? How could you communicate these reservations with your partner to ensure that every shared meal is a delight for both of you?

Mood and Setting the Scene
A Role-Playing or Desire Game!

Remember, mood and setting the scene are the canvas for your romantic escapades. Unleash your imagination, dare to explore uncharted territory, and create unforgettable moments that will deepen your bond and mutual desire.

- If you were to transform a room in your home into a sensual sanctuary for a night, which one would you choose, and how would you decorate it?

- Imagine you're in a movie. What kind of erotic scene would you like to film with your partner: a sensual dance at a masked ball, an adventure on a deserted beach, or perhaps a mysterious encounter on a night train?

- You and your partner have the opportunity to travel back in time for a night of love. What era would you choose, and how would you dress?

- If you had to choose a food item to play with and explore sensations on your partner's body, what would it be, and how would you use it?

- An unexpected bathroom leak requires the immediate intervention of a "plumber." How could this routine repair evolve into a wet and unexpected seduction game between you and your partner?

- You have the opportunity to gift your partner a fragrance that would instantly ignite your desire. What would be the key notes of this fragrance?

- If you were to surprise your partner with special lighting to set the mood for an intimate evening, would you opt for candles, soft lighting, lanterns, or perhaps string lights?

- You have the chance to whisk your partner away to an exotic location for a night. Where would you go, and what kind of adventure would you embark on?

- Before you lies a feather, a blindfold, and handcuffs. Which of these items would you like your partner to surprise you with, and how would you envision that scene?

- Picture your partner preparing a surprising striptease for you. What song would they choose to enchant you, and what clothing or accessory would they wear to add an unexpected final touch to their performance?

The Subtle Art of Caresses
Tell me what you like

Your bodies holds hidden treasures. Perhaps some less explored areas could become your new favorite spots for caresses?

- Imagine you are the tour guide of your own body. What are the points of interest (non-sexual) that you would recommend to your partner for a thorough exploration? Your neck? Your ears? Or perhaps your breasts, buttocks, inner thighs, back, belly, or feet?

- If you had to describe to your partner the ideal touch for these areas, how would you characterize it? Is it a gentle, firm, or lingering stroke? Do you prefer when they caress, kiss, lick, suck, gently nibble, scratch, or pinch you?

- When you think of an unforgettable caress, what part of your body immediately comes to mind?

- Let's continue exploring by focusing on your respective primary erogenous zones (genitals).

For you, Madam, do you reach cloud nine when your partner stimulates your clitoris? Vagina, G-spot or anus? Do you prefer when they caress you with their fingers, or perhaps with their penis, pubic area, a vibrating toy, or another accessory?

Now, gentlemen, it's your turn! What leaves you bedazzled? When she strokes your glans? The body of the penis, the testicles, or the anus? Do you prefer when she strokes you with her fingers, vulva, vagina, breasts, or maybe with an accessory?

- Conversely, are there areas that you would prefer your partner to approach with particular care or even avoid altogether during your intimate moments?

Getting Started
Exploring Cunnilingus and Fellatio

While oral sex can serve as an enticing prelude and sometimes even a delightful alternative to what's commonly known as "full intercourse," it should always remain a matter of choice. There are no absolutes in this practice! What truly matters is having a genuine desire to please each other.

- If your genitals were treats, what flavor would yours be, and how would you prefer your partner to savor it? Sucking, licking, or perhaps sensually nibbling and teasing with the tongue?

- When it comes to exploring oral caresses, are there any uncharted territories between you and your partner that spark your curiosity?

- Some view oral-genital games as a graceful dance of lips and tongue. What tempo do you both prefer: slow and sensual or lively and playful?

- How would you like to guide your partner to show them precisely what makes you ecstatic during cunnilingus or fellatio?

- Do you think there are ways to make these intimate moments even more special? Are there any subtle adjustments or novel ideas you'd like to experiment with?

- Just like a sommelier savoring wine, exploring oral-genital intimacy comes with its nuances. Are there any preferences or boundaries you'd like to set with your partner in this unique sphere?

Now that you've explored the intricacies of intimate communication, it's time to explore another equally potent form of expression—your bodies!

Did you really think this quiz was the boldest part of your journey? Think again and get ready to dive into the captivating world of Kamasutra positions, neatly categorized for your enjoyment (and perhaps a few chuckles) based on their level of difficulty. From tender positions to the most acrobatic, there's something to cater to every taste and flexibility.

But before you turn the page, remember: just like with our quiz, the aim isn't to try everything or achieve perfection, but to discover what truly excites you and your partner!

3
The Sex Position Guide
Sensual Warm-Up

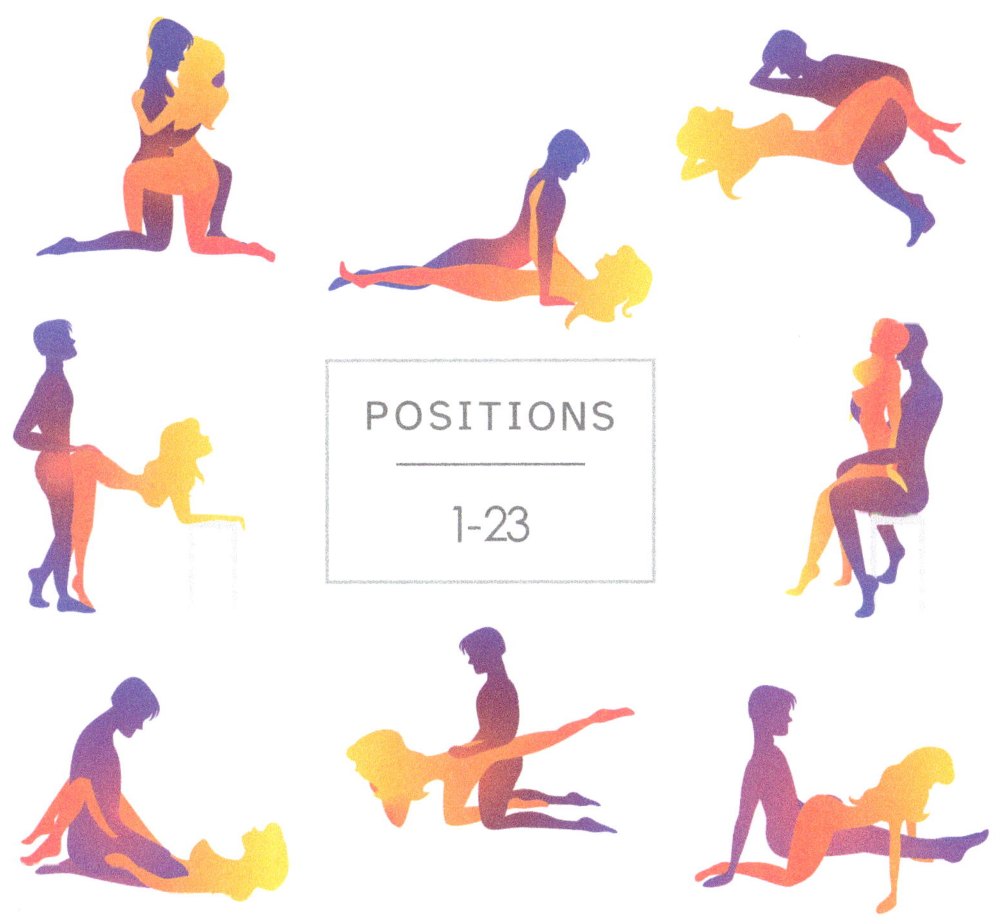

The Super 8:

In this position, the woman lies on her back with her legs extended and slightly apart. The man positions himself between her legs, somewhat like he's going to do push-ups, with his arms extended and hands placed on either side of her face.

The woman places her hands on her partner's hips and encourages him to trace figure eights inside her.

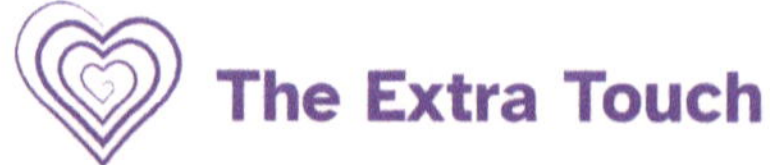 **The Extra Touch**

Placing a small cushion beneath the woman's buttocks allows for deeper penetration and heightened stimulation the G-spot.

The Super 8

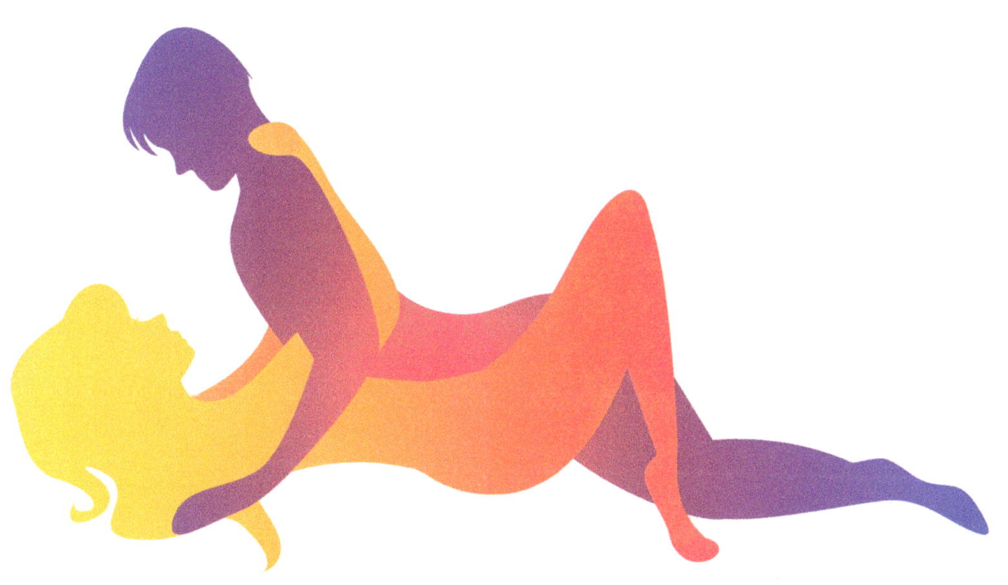

2

The Thigh Master:

The man lies on his back with bent legs and knees pointing upward. The woman straddles him, facing away. She then lowers herself to allow penetration while firmly gripping her partner's knees. The woman's abdomen is close to the man's bent knees, providing support for rocking back and forth and performing up-and-down movements.

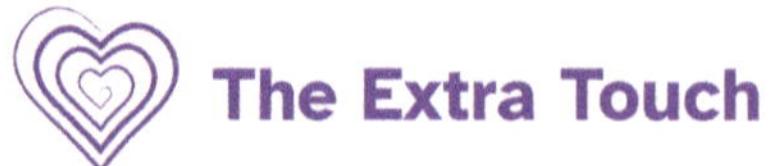 **The Extra Touch**

In this position, the partners can't see each other, allowing them to focus entirely on their sensations! The man enjoys a splendid view of his partner's buttocks and can admire her as she takes charge.

The Thigh Master

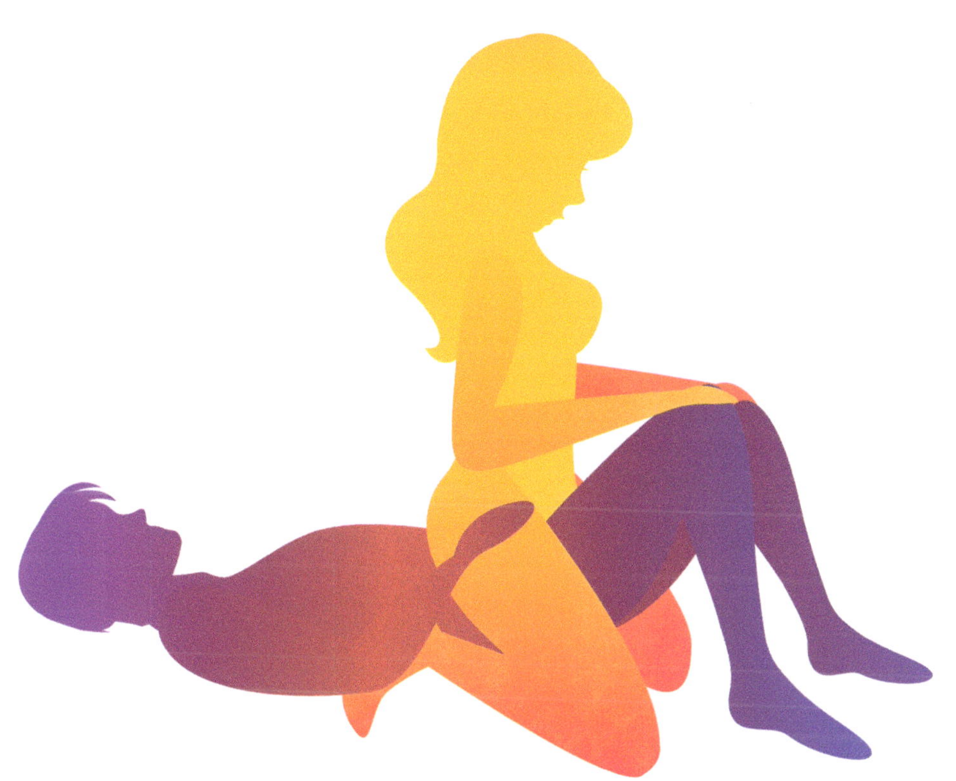

3

The Kneel:

The partners kneel face to face. The woman spreads her legs and glides them on either side of her partner's. She lifts her pelvis and positions herself against her partner. The man advances one knee between the woman's legs and penetrates her.

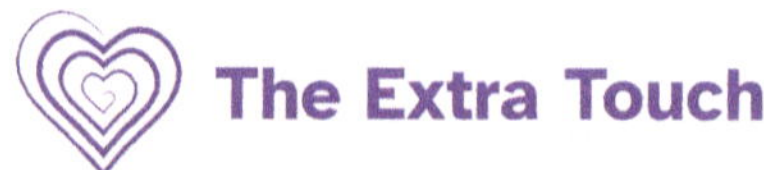 **The Extra Touch**

This position is ideal for kissing, locking intense gazes, sharing tender whispers, or indulging in intimate caresses to intensify sensations.

The Kneel

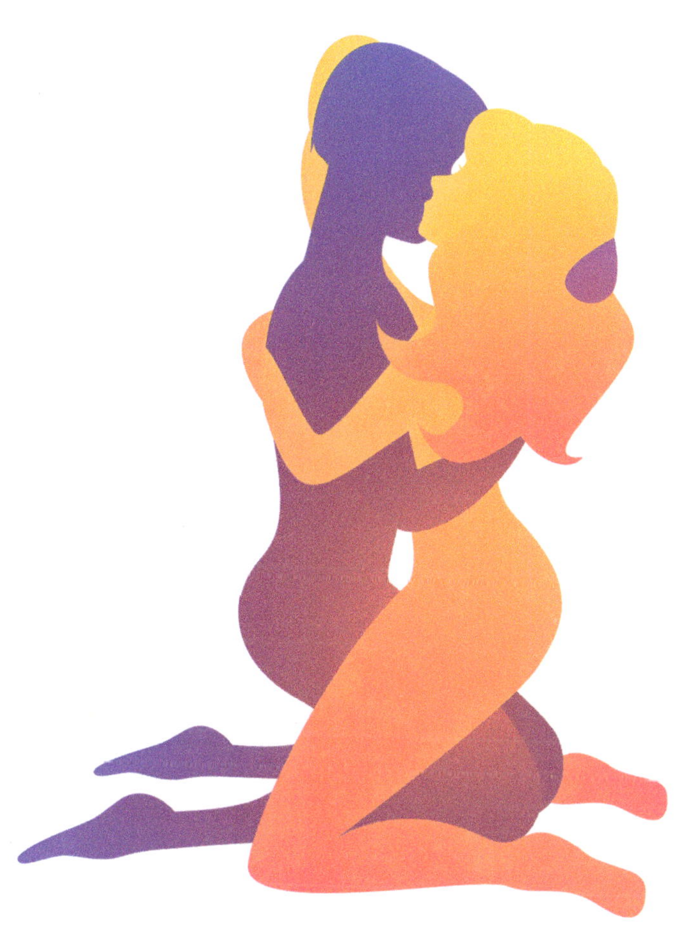

4

The Close-Up:

The partners lie side by side, spooning, with the man behind the woman. The woman presses her pelvis against the man's and ensnares his legs between hers. In this position, penetration is gentle, as the man's movements are restricted. However, he can lavish his partner with neck kisses and fondle her breasts or clitoris.

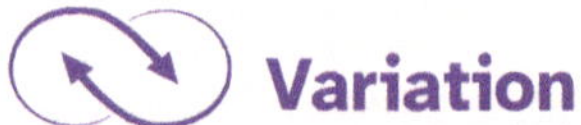 **Variation**

By extending their legs, the partners transition into the spooning position. The 99 and spooning are perfect for pregnant women or for experimenting with anal intercourse.

The Close-Up

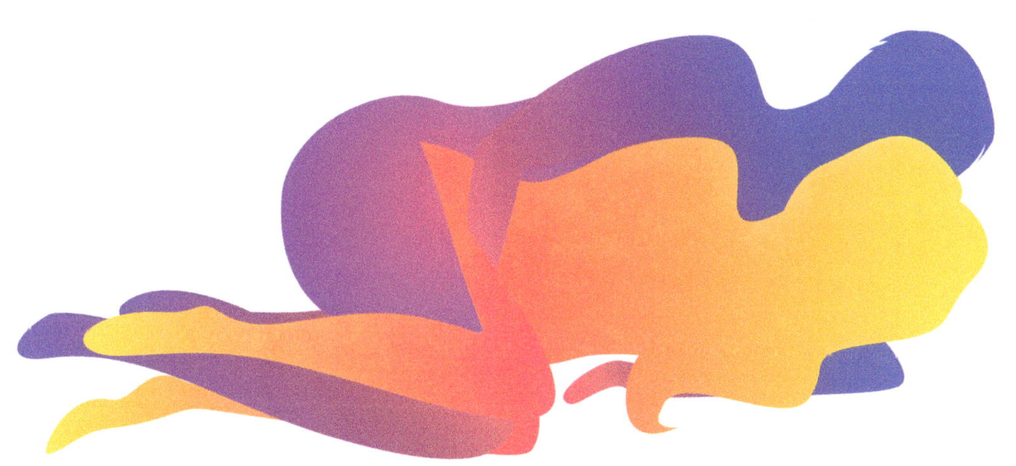

The Kneeling Wheelbarrow:

The woman gets on all fours, supporting herself on her forearms. The man kneels and positions himself behind her. He lifts one of her legs horizontally to facilitate penetration. In this position, the man controls the rhythm.

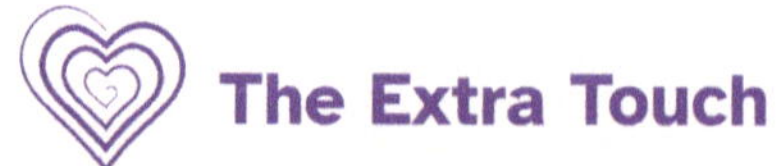 **The Extra Touch**

For added comfort, the partner can place her leg on a low table or stool and her forearms on a cushion.

The Kneeling Wheelbarrow

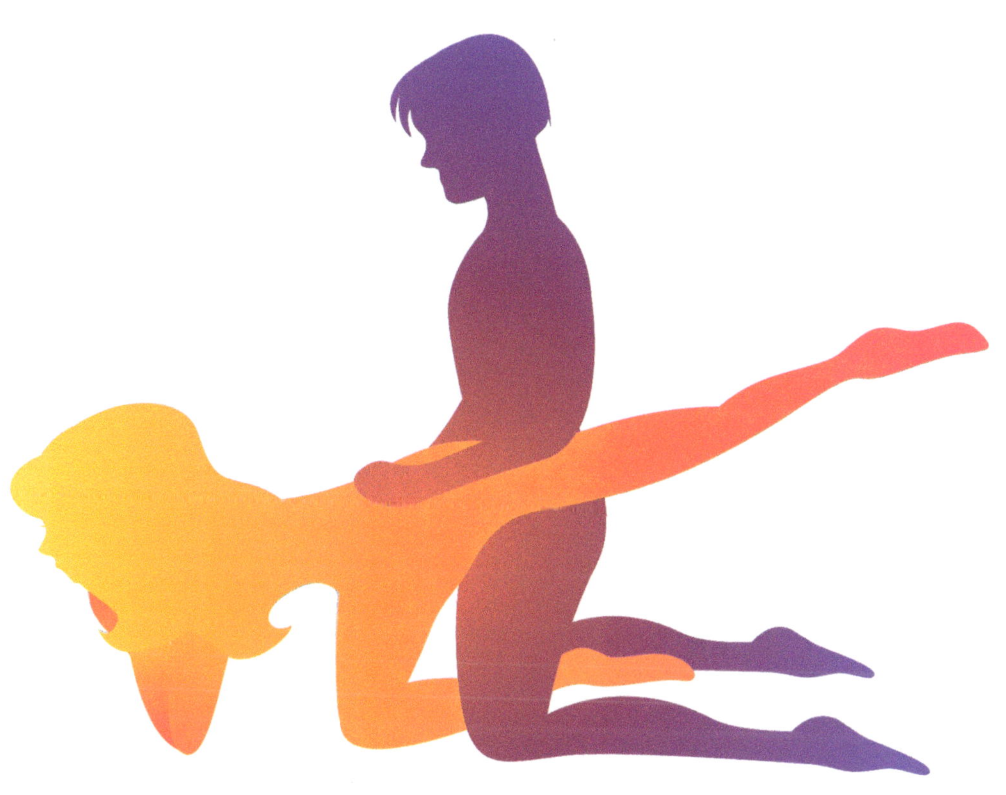

6

The Zen Pause:

The partners lie facing each other on their sides. The man has one leg extended and the other bent upward. The woman places her leg over his waist.

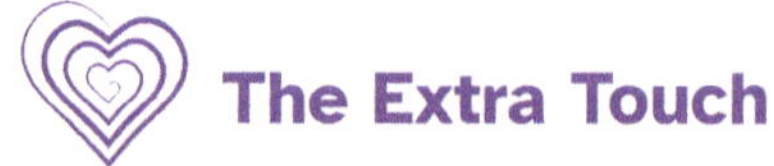 **The Extra Touch**

This is the perfect position to take a break when the couple is on the brink of orgasm.

The Zen Pause

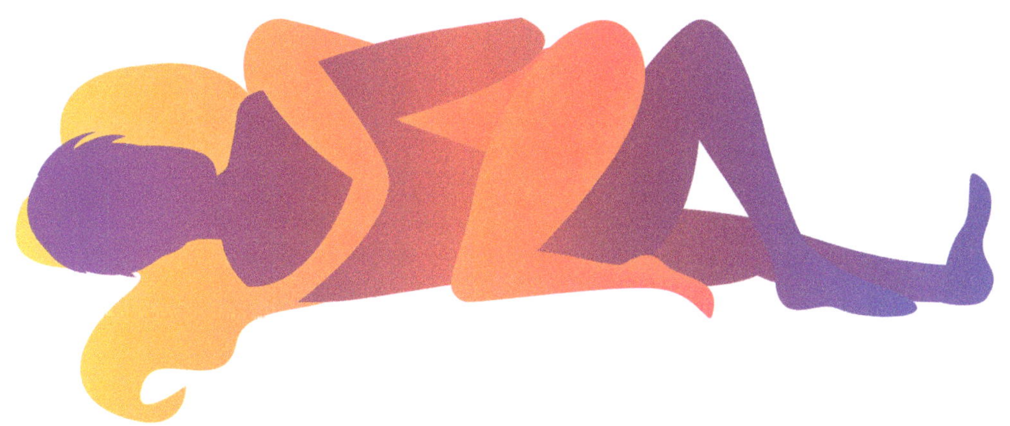

7

The Side Saddle:

The man lies on his back with his legs slightly apart. The woman positions herself on top, with her legs perpendicular to his and her arms resting at the back.

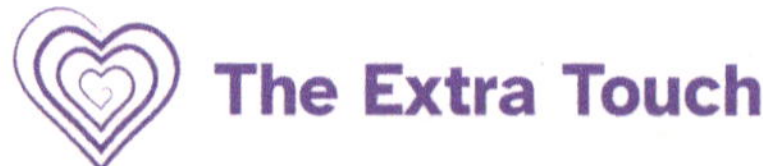 **The Extra Touch**

By adjusting the space between her thighs, the woman can control the depth of penetration. In this position, she can also caress her partner's scrotum.

The Side Saddle

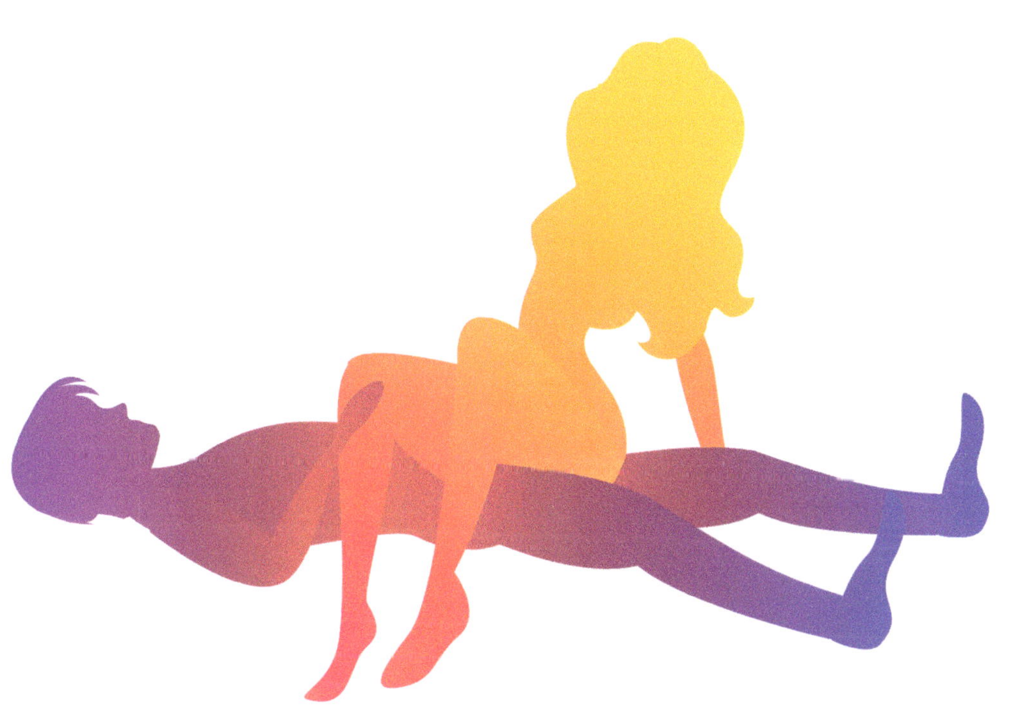

The Amazon:

The man sits on a chair or on the edge of the bed. The woman straddles him, making sure her feet touch the ground to facilitate back-and-forth movements.

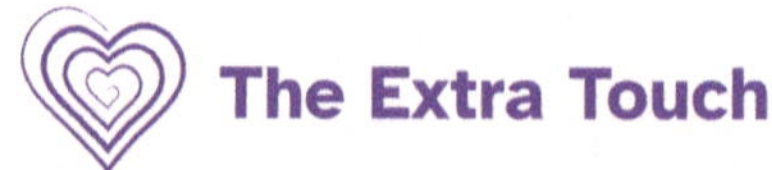 **The Extra Touch**

Ideal Position After a Sensual Strip Tease.

The Amazon

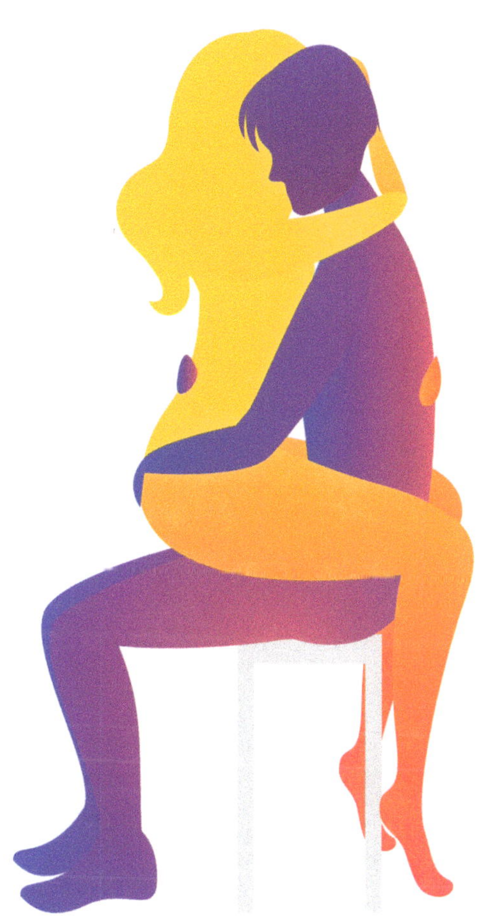

9

The Nirvana:

The woman lies flat on her back, extending her arms behind her head, gripping the headboard or placing her hands on the wall. The man then stretches out on top of her. As he begins to penetrate, the woman contracts her muscles and tightens her thighs, pushing firmly against the wall.

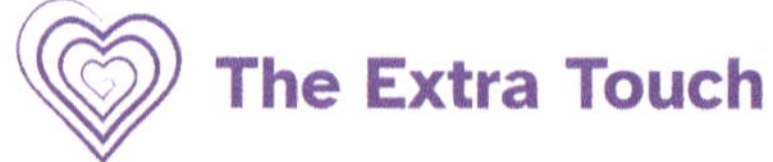 **The Extra Touch**

The man can also extend his arms, intertwining his hands with the woman's for an even more sensual embrace.

The Nirvana

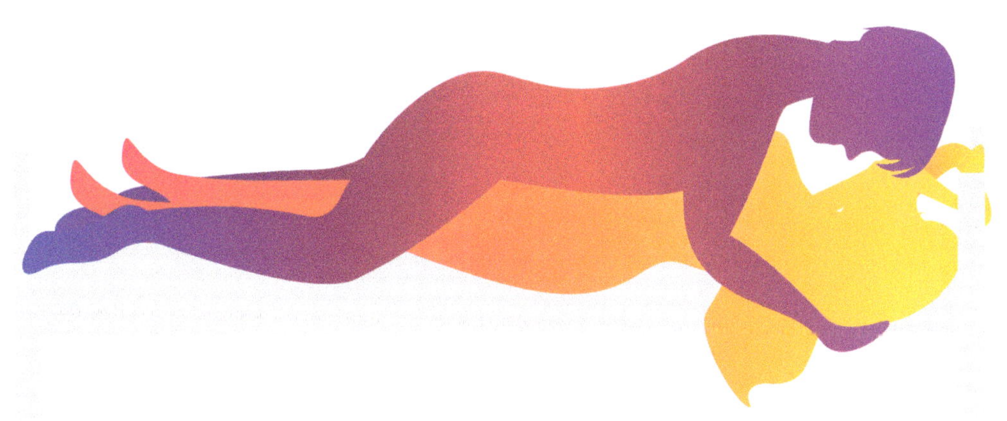

Afternoon Delight:

The woman lies on her back with her legs bent. The man stretches out on his side, perpendicular to her. His legs are extended beneath hers, aligning his pelvis with her buttocks. With one hand, he supports his head, while the other is free to roam his partner's body. The woman, too, has both hands free. She can use them as pillows or take the opportunity to caress her lover's body or her own!

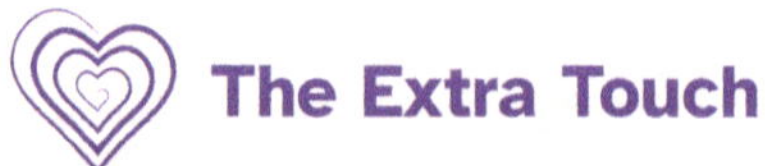 **The Extra Touch**

Perfect for those days when you're tired! A comfortable position that doesn't require much effort and allows for a delightful moment of pleasure while relaxing.

Afternoon Delight

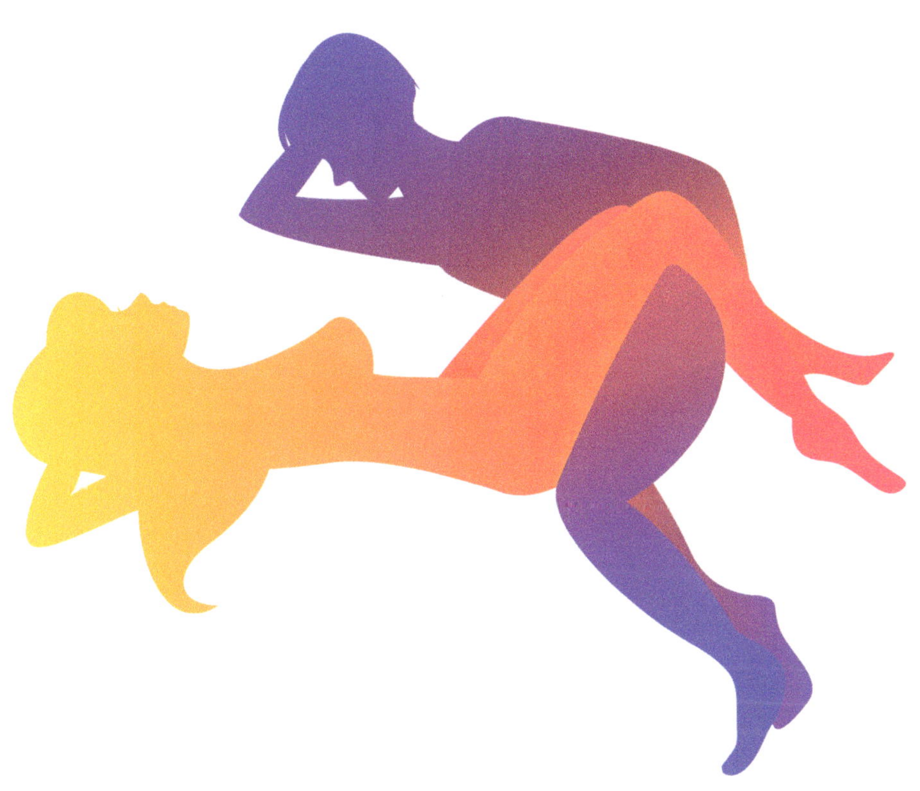

11

The Visitor:

Partners stand facing each other. The woman places one of her legs between her lover's. The man pulls her close, holding her buttocks firmly with one or both hands while she embraces him. The man can easily stimulate his partner with his own, and even penetrate if desired.

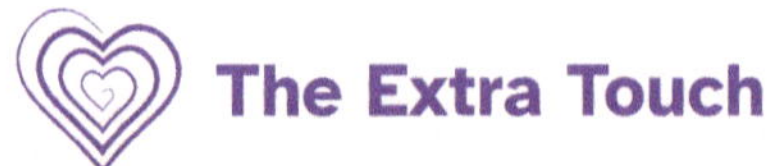 **The Extra Touch**

Penetration is usually shallow and often requires the woman to elevate herself, either by wearing heels or standing on a platform.

The Visitor

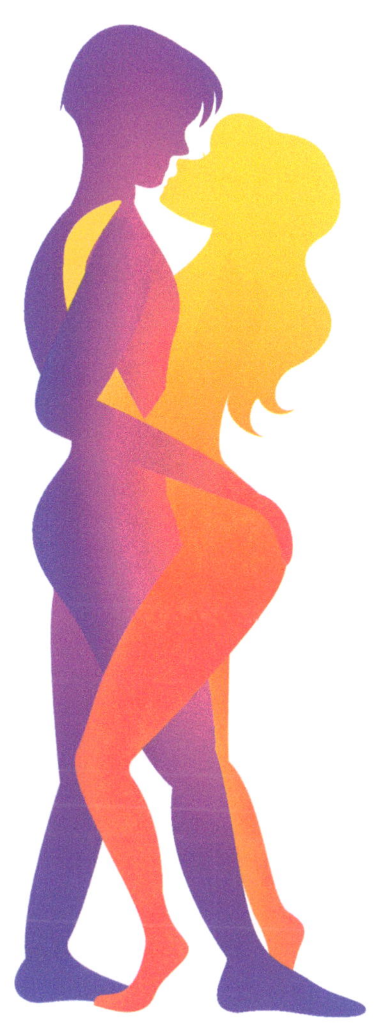

12

The Reverse Cowgirl:

The man lies on his back with his legs extended. The woman straddles him, facing away, while kneeling. She initiates back-and-forth movements, using her hands for support on the bed or her partner's legs. If desired, the man can accompany her movements by using his hands on her hips.

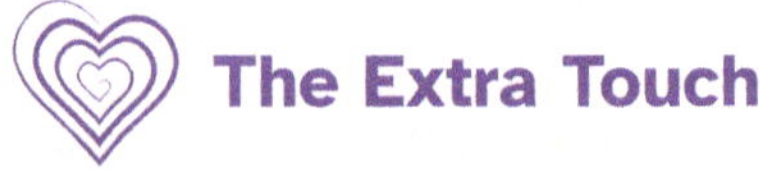 **The Extra Touch**

To spice up this position, the woman can caress her partner's inner thighs or even his genitals. A word of caution: avoid going too vigorously, as the angle requires finesse.

The Reverse Cowgirl

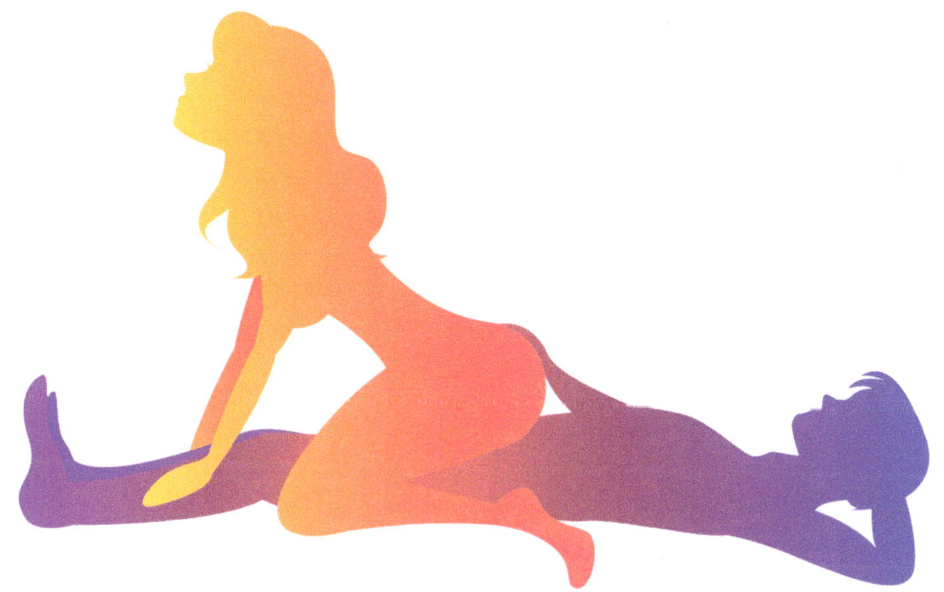

13

The Whisper:

The woman and the man lie side by side, facing each other. She lifts her legs, wrapping them around her partner's waist and clasping him.

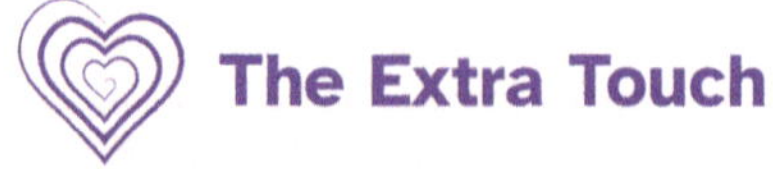 **The Extra Touch**

A deeply intimate position that allows partners to whisper sweet nothings, caress each other, and share passionate gazes.

The Whisper

42

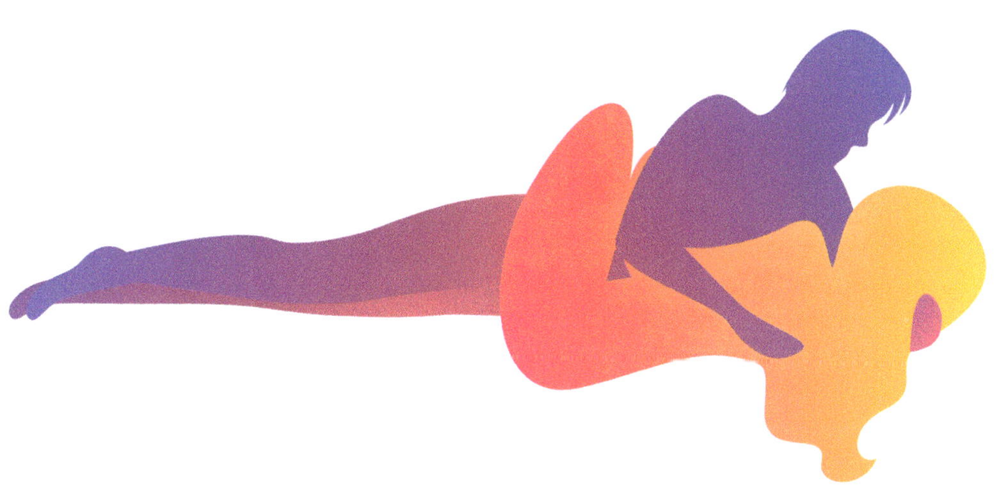

14

The Stair Master:

The woman kneels on one step of a staircase, using a higher step for support. Her partner stands behind her, holding her hips for penetration. For added comfort, he can also kneel on a step.

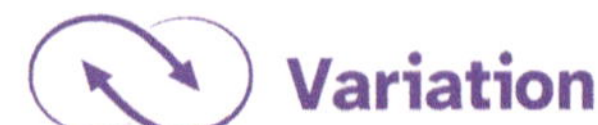 **Variation**

If both partners enjoy a challenge, they can decide to climb the steps one by one during the act, reaching new heights of pleasure!

The Stair Master

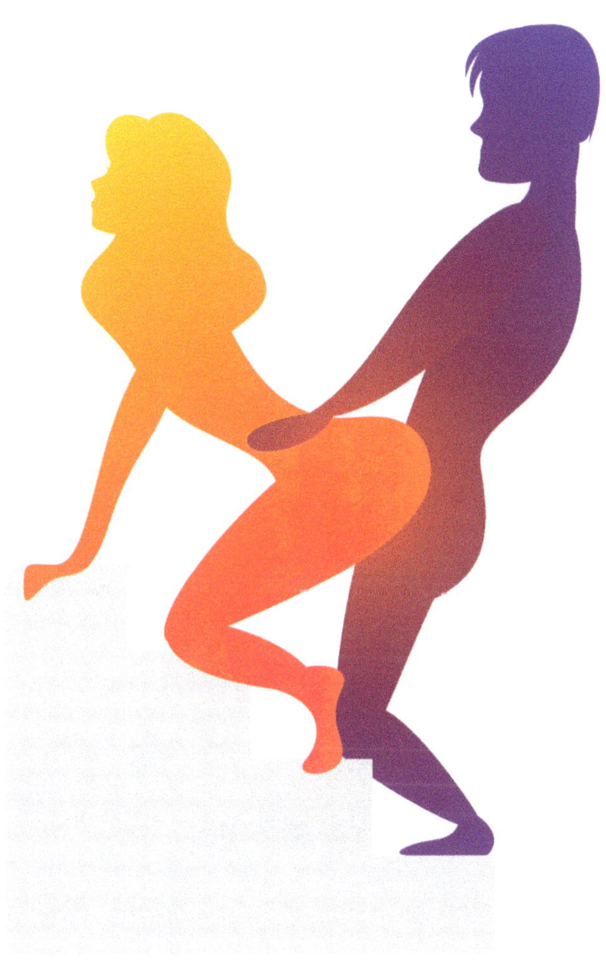

The Classic:

Also known as the classic position. The woman lies on her back, thighs slightly apart, and the man lies on top, at the right height for penetration.

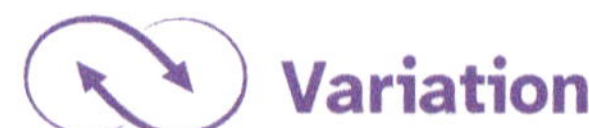 **Variation**

The missionary dance: The woman slightly bends her legs, spreads them, uses her feet for support, and makes rhythmic movements with her pelvis.

The Classic

46

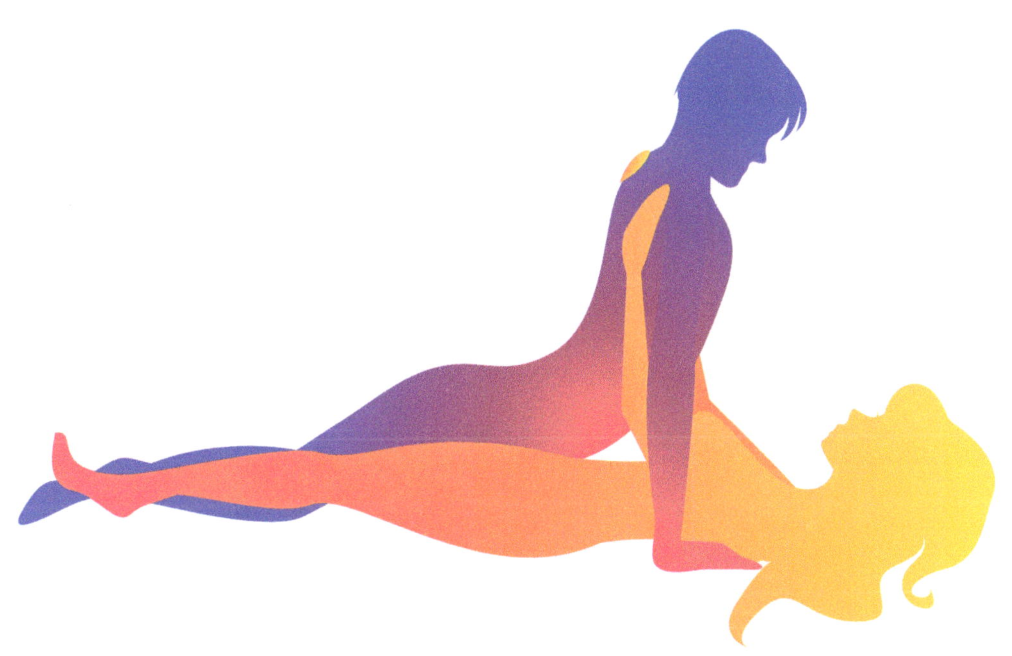

The Proposal:

The man and the woman kneel face to face. Their respective feet are placed on opposite sides. They gently move back and forth to facilitate penetration.

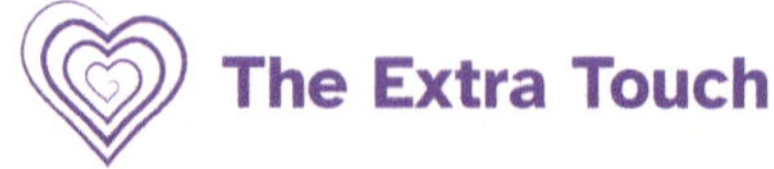 **The Extra Touch**

One of the most tender positions, allowing partners to stay embraced throughout intercourse and caress each other from head to buttocks.

The Proposal

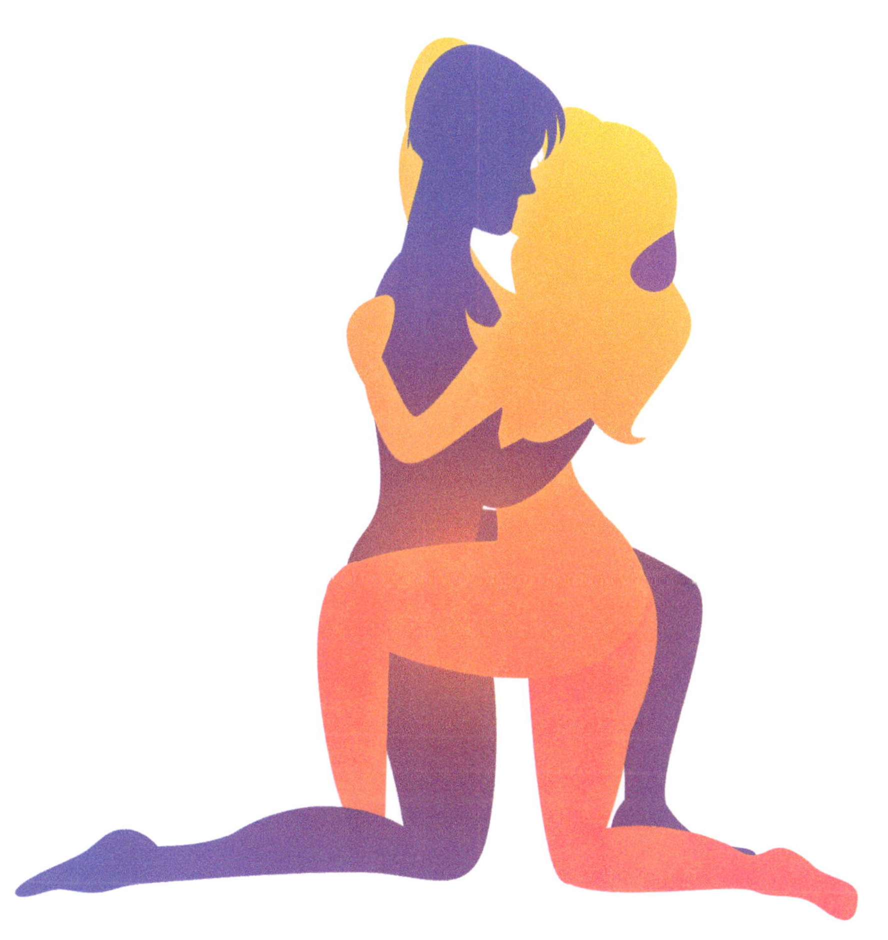

The Slide:

The man lies on his back, and his partner, with her legs slightly apart, lies flat on her stomach on top of him. While he can make gentle movements with his pelvis, it's the woman who controls the depth and pace of penetration.

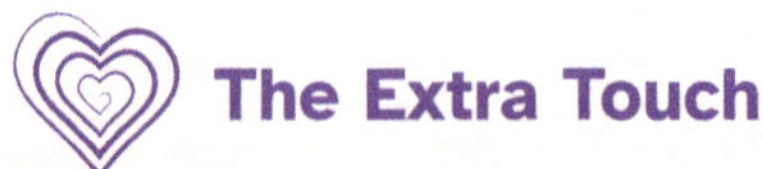 **The Extra Touch**

In this position, the woman takes the lead. With his free hands, the man can explore her back and buttocks, while the sensation of her chest against his intensifies desire.

The Slide

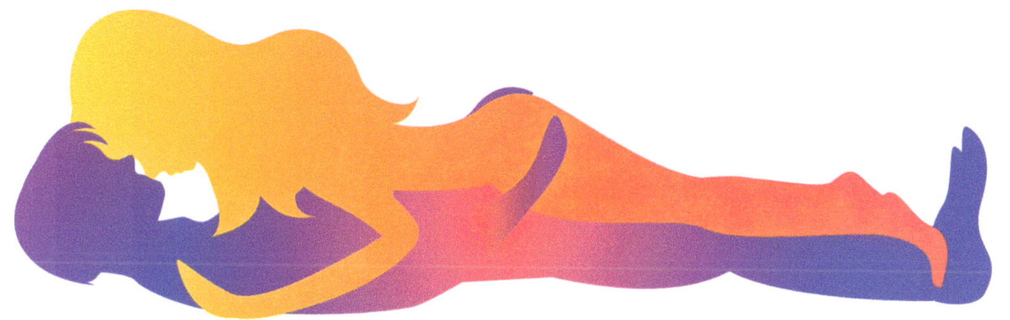

18

Doggy Style:

One of the most famous Kamasutra positions. The woman gets on all fours, supporting herself with her hands. The man kneels behind her and penetrates at a pace that suits him. To enhance his partner's pleasure, he can caress her thighs, buttocks, back, breasts, or clitoris. Depending on the width of her legs, the woman can adjust the depth of penetration.

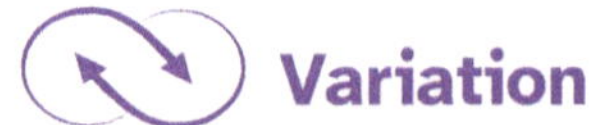 **Variation**

The woman is on all fours at the edge of the bed, and the man enters her from behind while standing on the floor.

Doggy Style

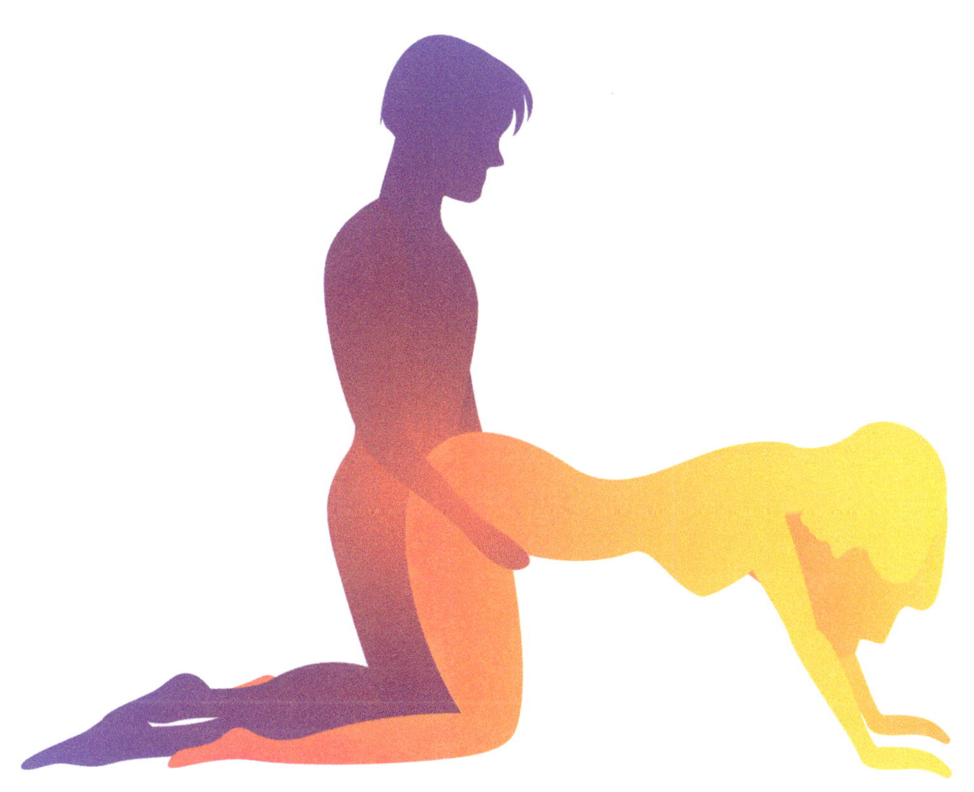

19

The Perch:

The man sits with his legs slightly apart. His partner straddles him, ensuring her feet touch the ground. She can then move up and down using her legs and lean forward or backward to vary the penetration angle. The man can take advantage of this position to caress her neck, breasts, and clitoris.

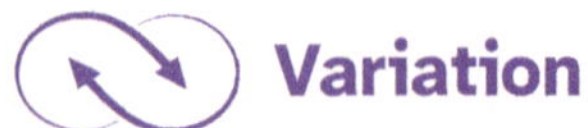 **Variation**

To change the penetration angle, the woman can lean fully forward and use the ground for support, placing her hands on it.

The Perch

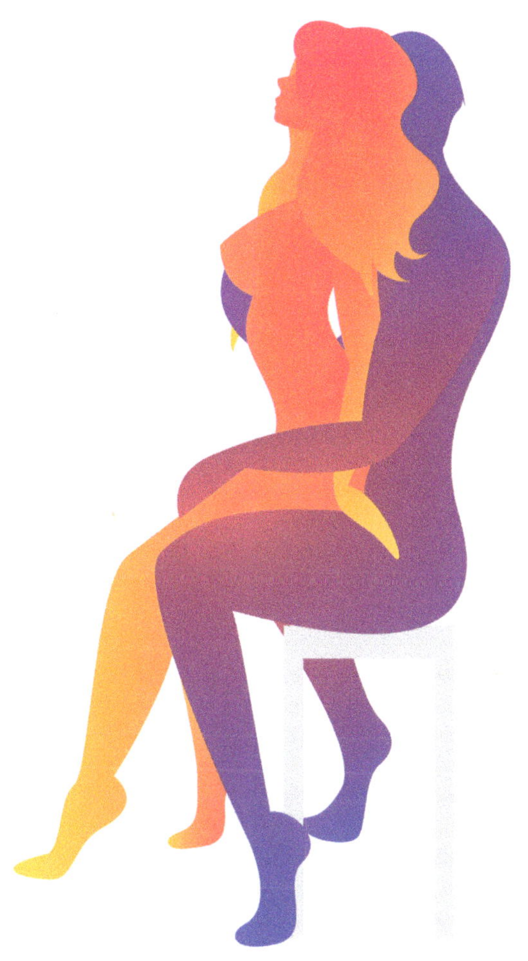

20

The Galley:

The man is seated with his legs extended. To maintain balance, he can place his hands behind him or lean against a wall or the bedframe. The woman straddles him while kneeling with her back to him. Leaning forward, she initiates back-and-forth movements, managing penetration depth and rhythm.

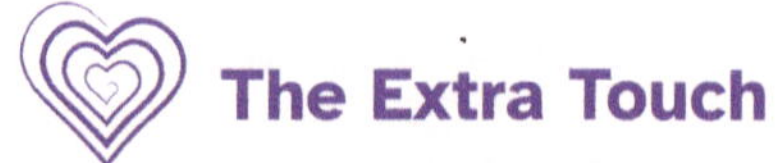

The Extra Touch

The man has an excellent view of his partner's buttocks and can admire her as she takes the lead.

The Galley

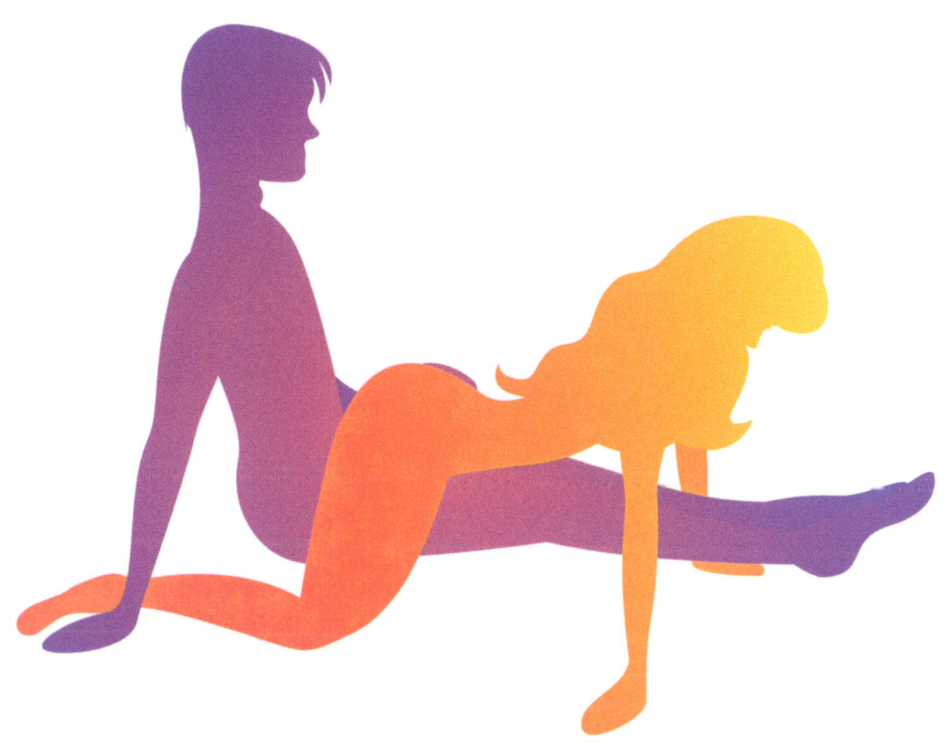

21

The Magic Mountain:

This position is similar to doggy style but more comfortable. The woman kneels and rests her upper body on a low table, couch, or a stack of pillows. The man kneels behind her, fitting perfectly with his chest against her back. She gently spreads her legs to allow penetration.

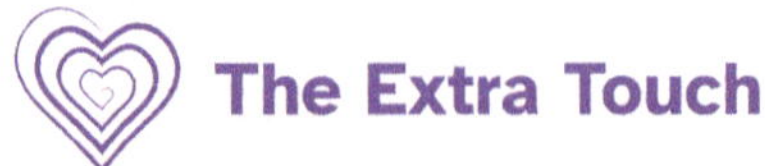 **The Extra Touch**

Here, there's no domination, but rather a communion perfect for kisses and caresses. A genuine body-to-body experience, fostering intimacy and sensuality.

The Magic Mountain

58

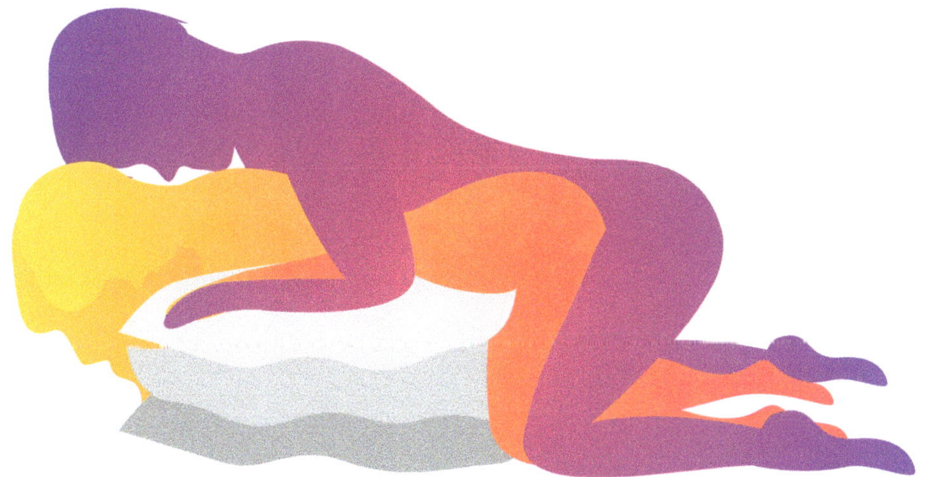

22

Wide Opened:

The man kneels, and the woman lies across his knees, wrapping her legs around him. In this position, the man manages penetration and chooses the rhythm, while the woman can still facilitate movements by slightly pushing back with her pelvis.

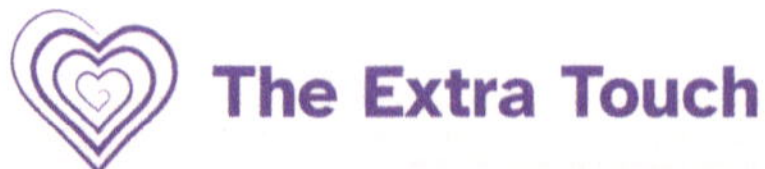 **The Extra Touch**

The woman surrenders entirely to her partner, who can enhance her pleasure by caressing her breasts and clitoris. An ideal position for pregnant women.

Wide Opened

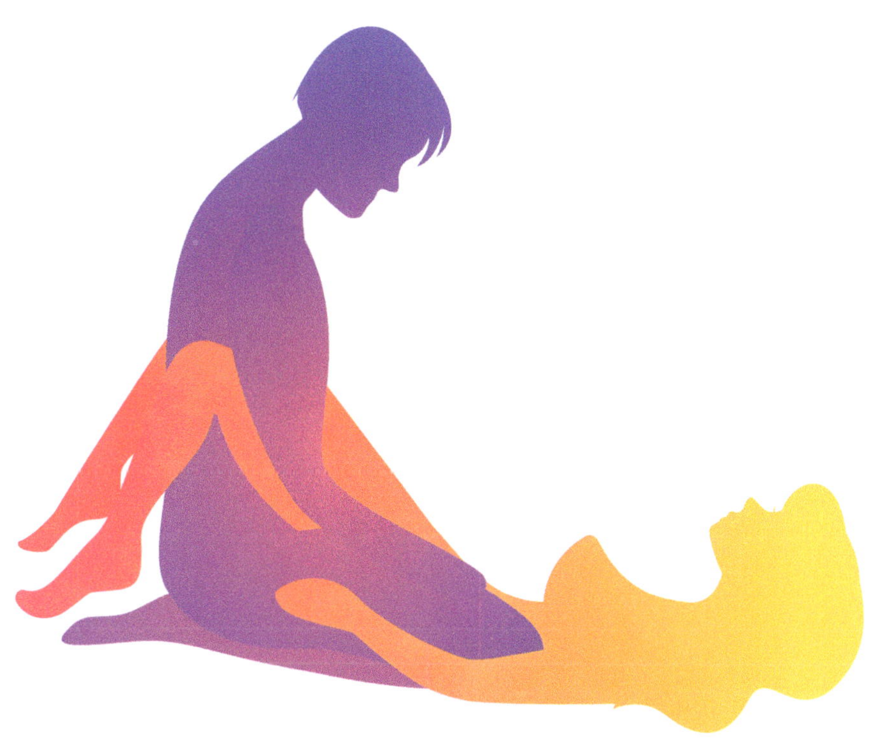

23

The Fan:

The woman rests her forearms on a chair, stool, or armchair, offering her posterior to her partner. The man stands behind her for penetration. He determines the pace of thrusting. His hands are entirely free to caress her erogenous zones, including her breasts, buttocks, inner thighs, and more!

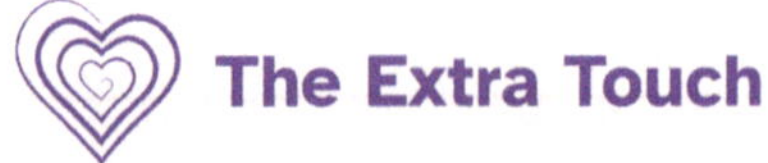 **The Extra Touch**

Use a higher or lower support to vary the penetration angle and sensations.

The Fan

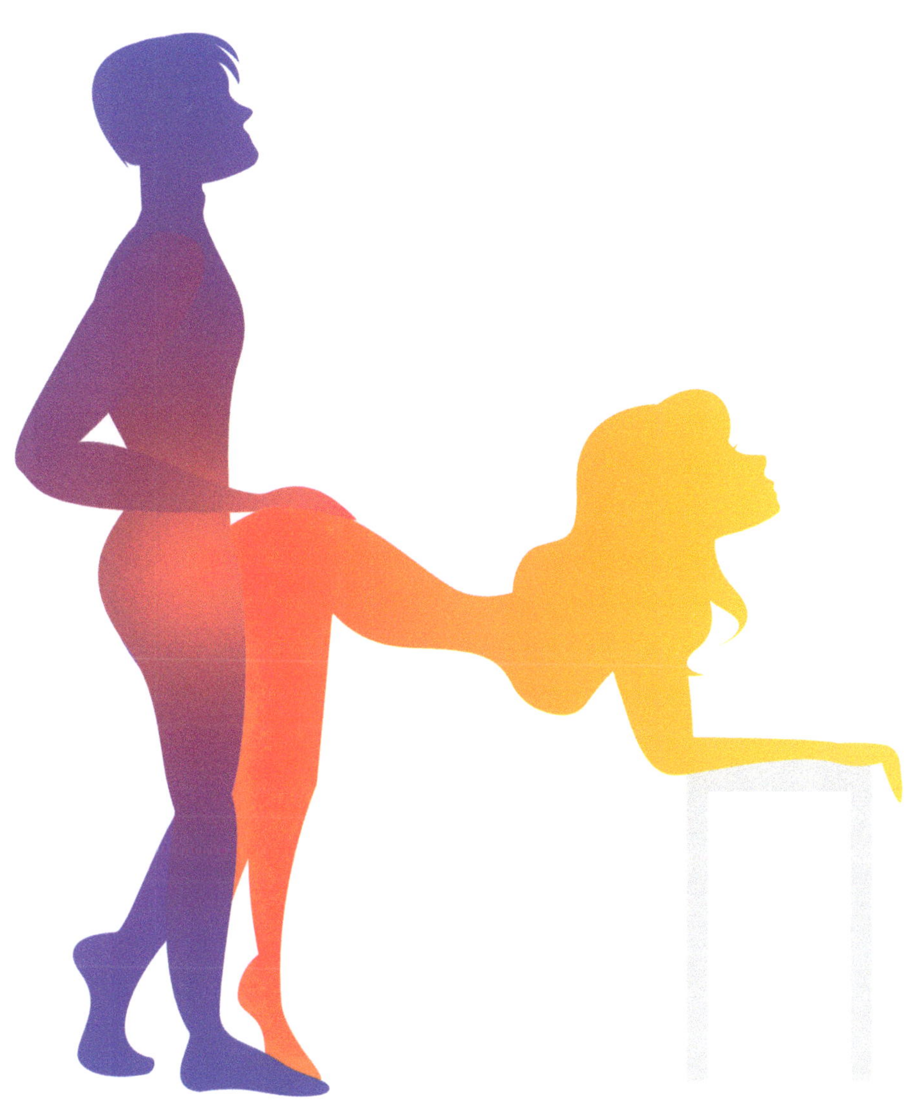

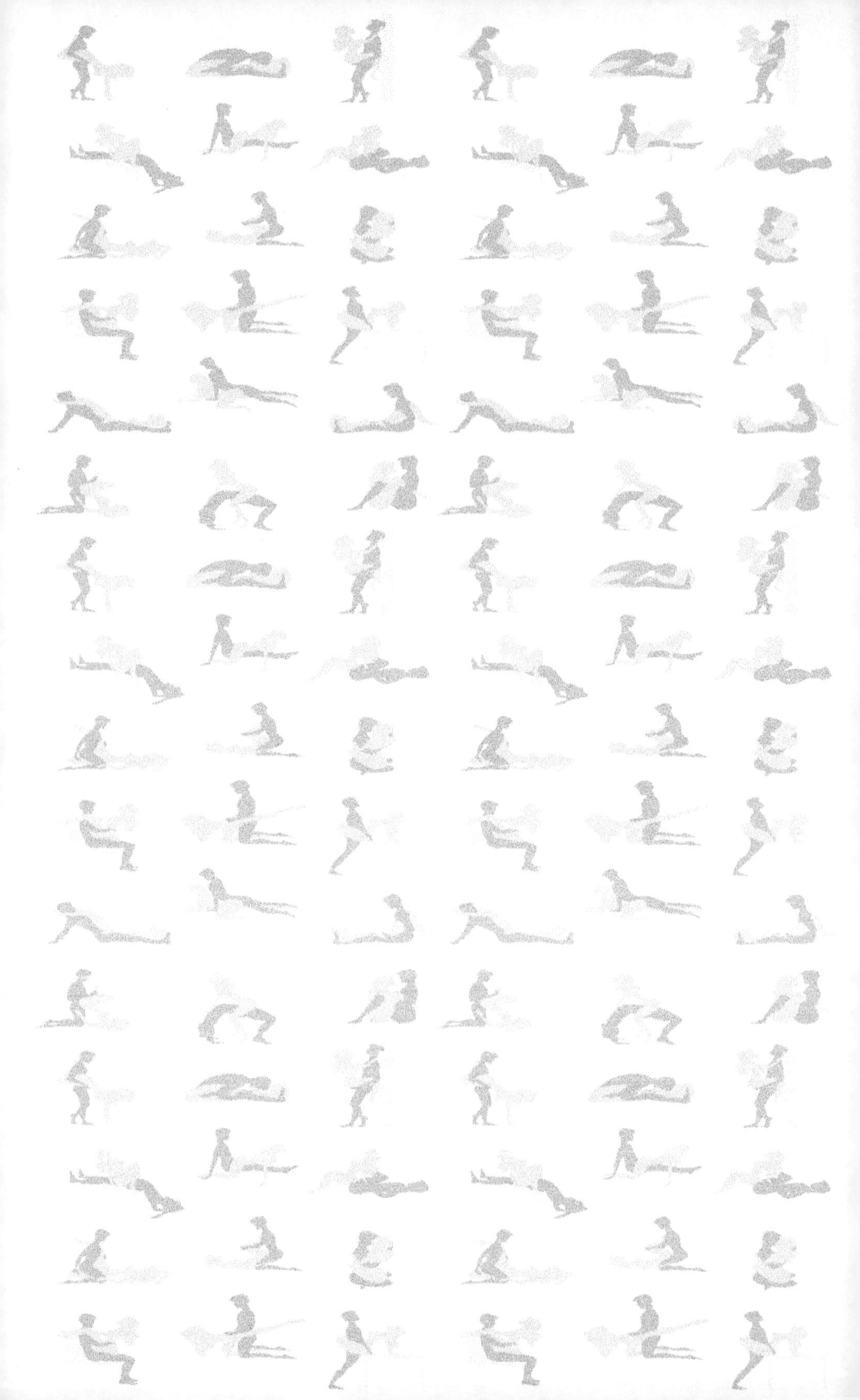

Sizzling Adventures

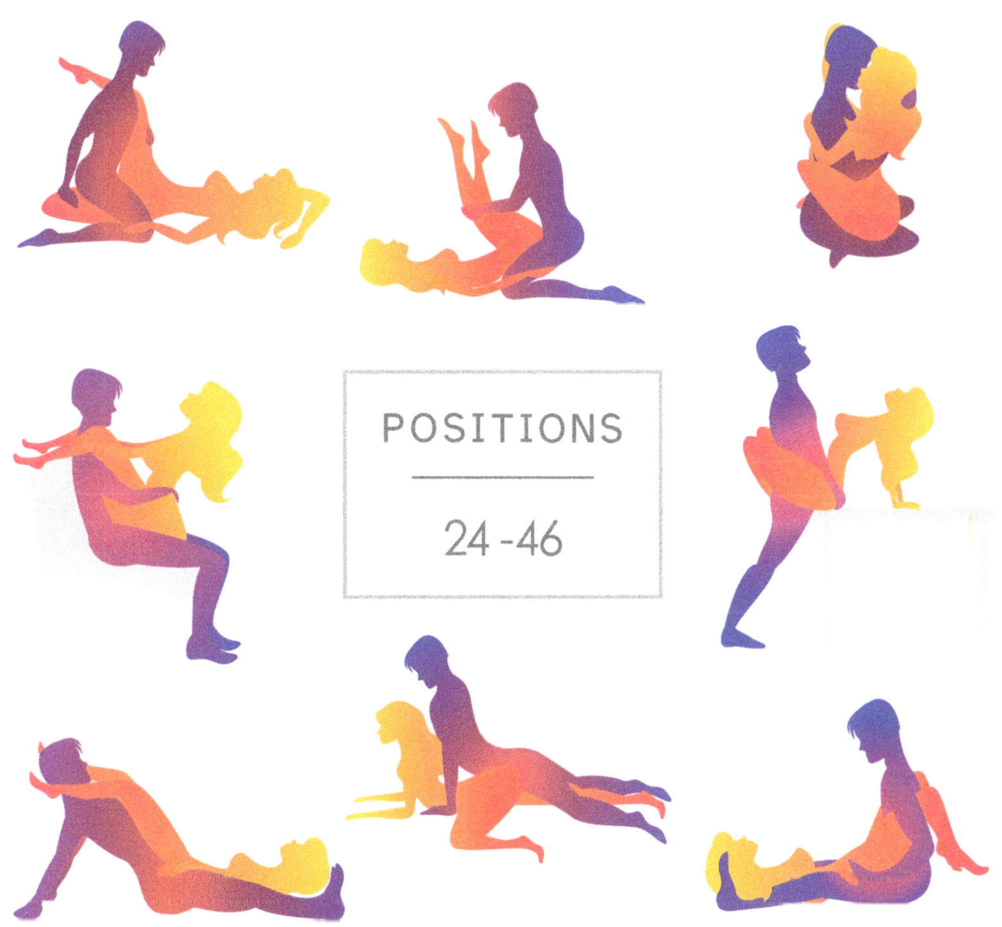

24

Indrani:

The woman lies on her back, legs drawn up to her chest. The man kneels, positioning himself at her level. Once in position, she places her feet on his chest or under his armpits. For added stability, the woman can grip the man's thighs, while he holds onto her hips or knees.

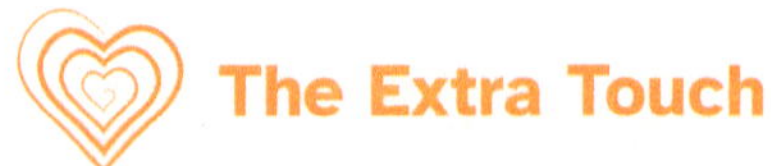

The Extra Touch

The woman's buttocks should be slightly elevated to make penetration possible. For more comfort, a cushion can be placed under her lower back.

Indrani

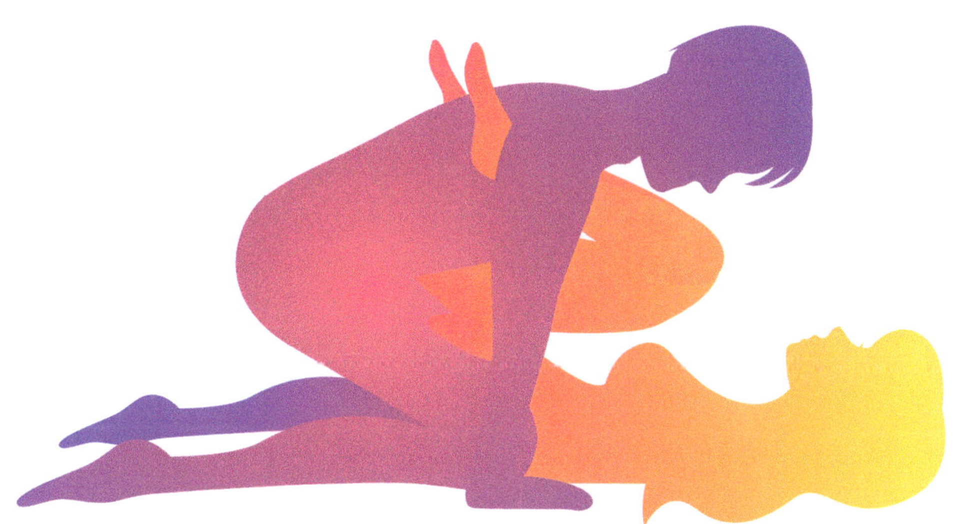

25

The Sphinx:

The woman lies on her stomach, lifting her upper body and resting on her forearms. One leg is bent, the other is extended. The man positions himself between her legs, supporting himself on his outstretched arms.

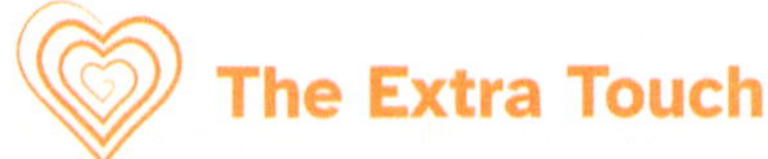 **The Extra Touch**

This creates an intense embrace, which can be comfortably enjoyed on the floor with the use of a thick mat.

The Sphinx

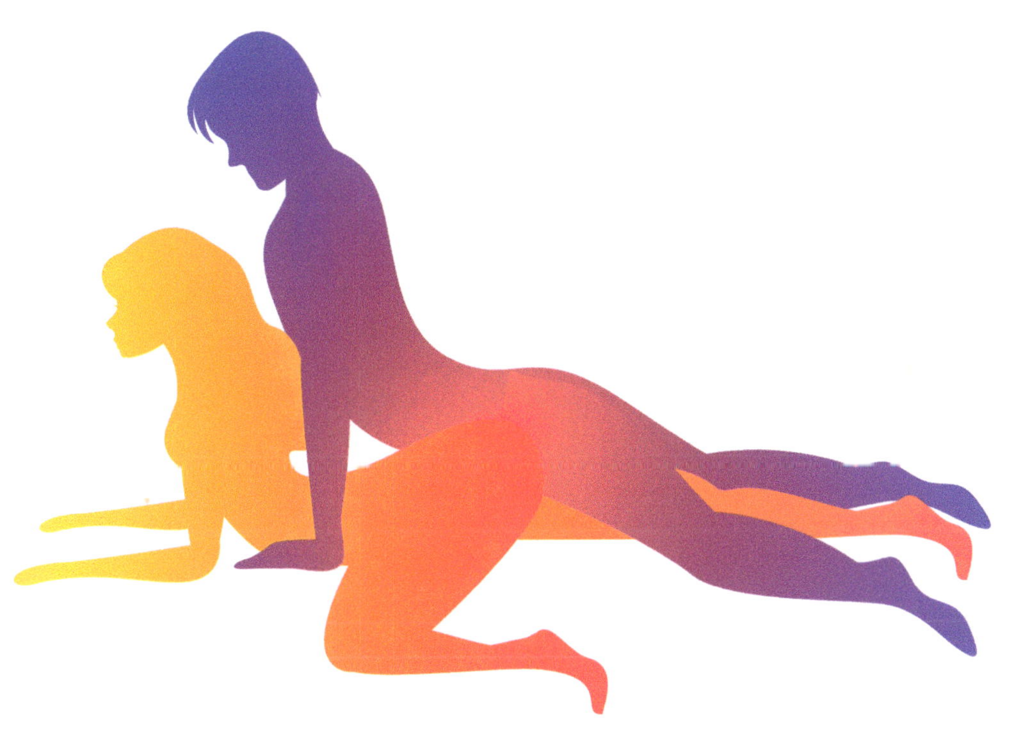

26

The Ship:

The man lies on his back. The woman sits on top of him, legs to the side and thighs apart. She takes the lead, gently making circular movements.

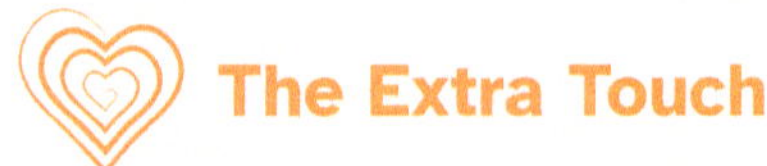 **The Extra Touch**

This position offers a different angle and allows stimulation of a new side of the man's pleasure. With his hands free, he can caress her back, thighs, buttocks, breasts, or clitoris at will.

The Ship

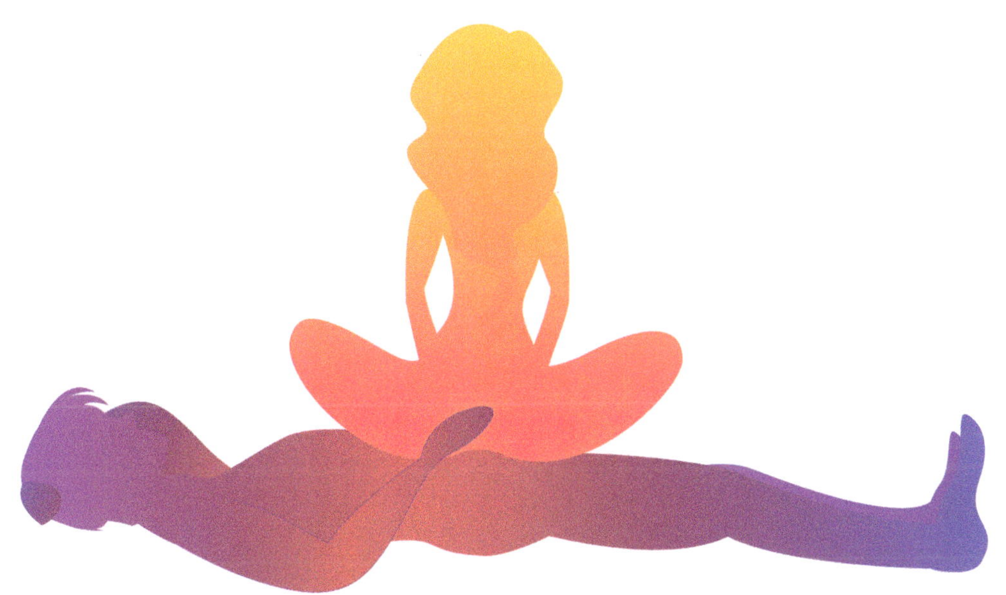

27

The Seated Ball:

The man is seated with slightly bent legs. The woman sits on his lap, leaning slightly forward to allow penetration. The man holds her by the waist, leaning in as well.

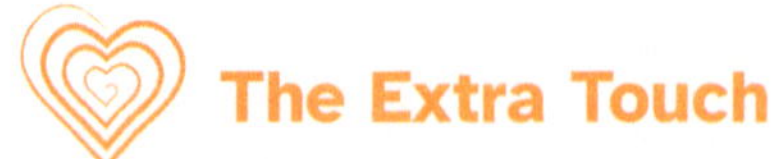 **The Extra Touch**

Partners can caress each other mutually. The penetration angle is ideal for intense sensations and achieving orgasm.

The Seated Ball

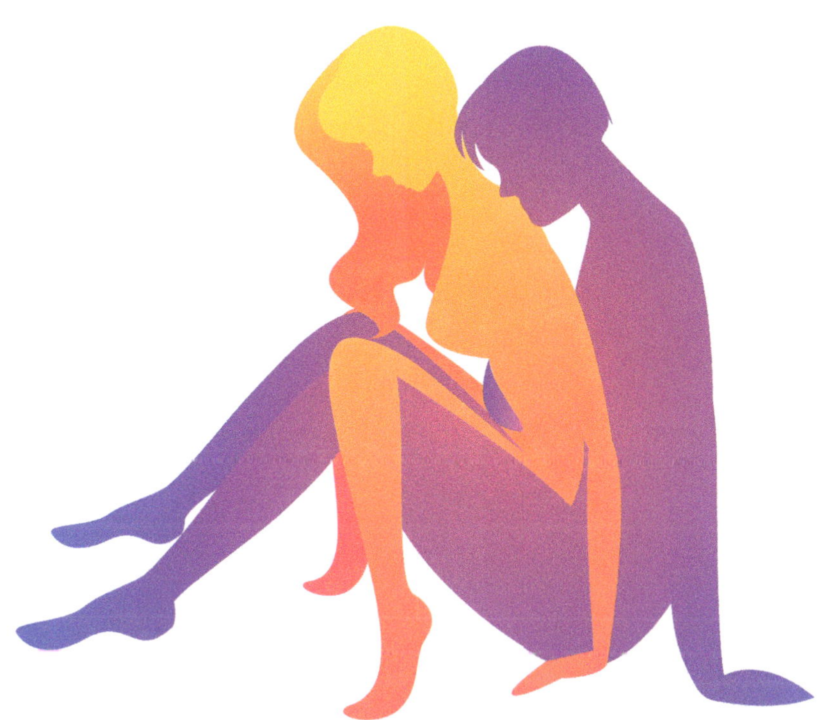

28

The Eagle:

The woman lies on her back, legs straight and raised vertically. The man positions himself facing her, spreading his knees and holding her ankles. For more comfort, a small flat cushion can be placed under the woman's buttocks.

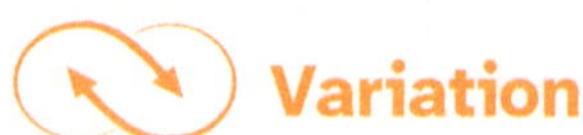 **Variation**

The woman lifts her pelvis off the bed and brings her knees as close to her chest as possible, becoming a sort of living pivot point that the man can gently rock to adjust penetration.

The Eagle

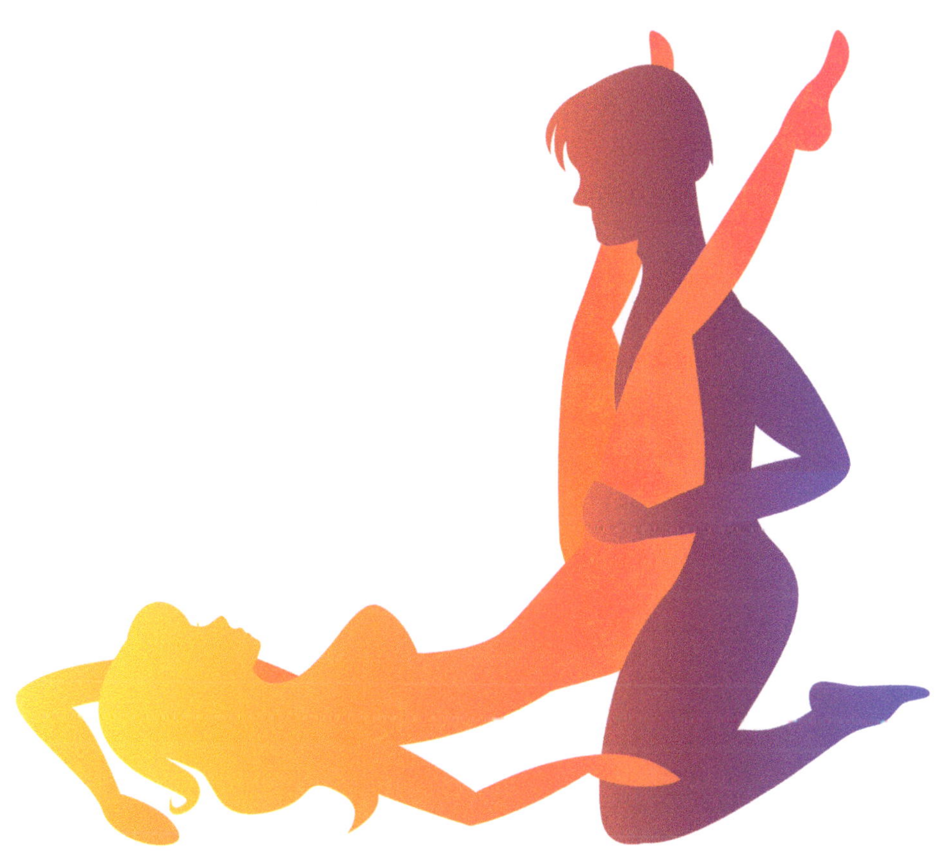

29

The Peg:

Partners lie on their sides, facing each other, with their faces in opposite directions. The woman snuggles against the man, enveloping his legs with her arms and thighs.

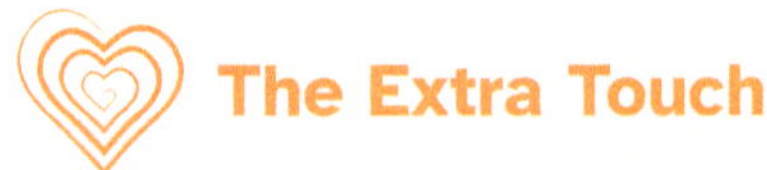 **The Extra Touch**

This position provides a different angle of penetration than usual and offers an exciting view of the partner's buttocks. The man can easily caress her lower back, thighs, buttocks, or anus.

The Peg

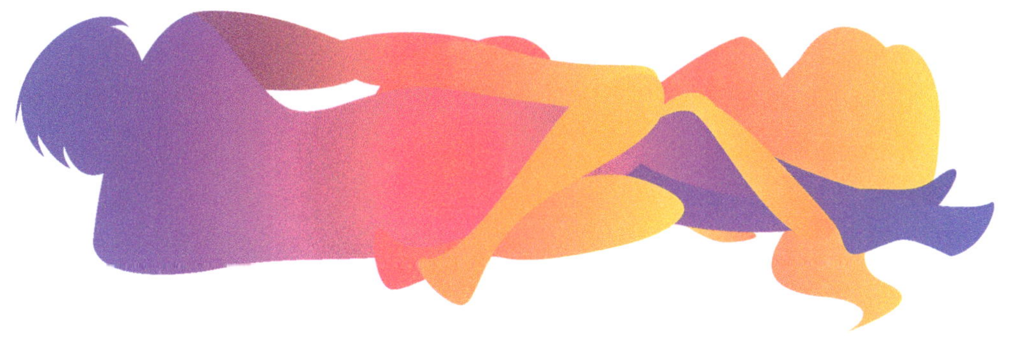

The Glowing Juniper:

The man is seated, legs extended in front of him and slightly apart. The woman lies on her back between his legs, placing her thighs around his chest. He lifts her pelvis and holds her by the hips to control the rhythm of penetration.

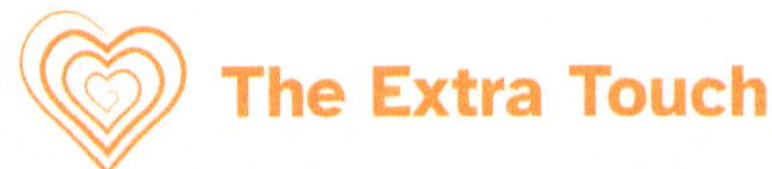 **The Extra Touch**

In this position, the woman can caress her clitoris, offering an arousing spectacle to her partner. The man can also lean forward to kiss her breasts.

The Glowing Juniper

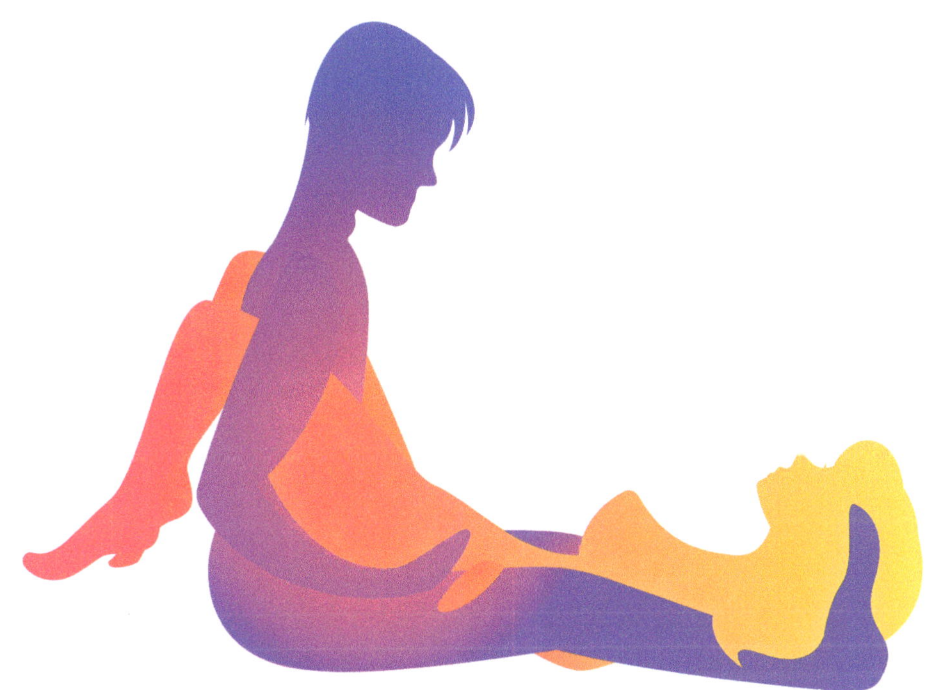

31

The Hinge:

The man is kneeling, thighs slightly apart. He leans back, supporting himself on his outstretched arms. The woman positions herself on all fours, facing away from him. She sets the rhythm for penetration.

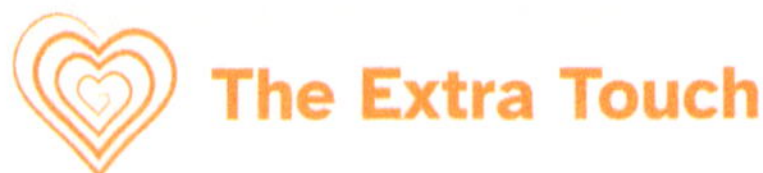 **The Extra Touch**

This is a very exciting position for the partner, as it provides a magnificent view of his companion's buttocks, allowing him to completely surrender to her.

The Hinge

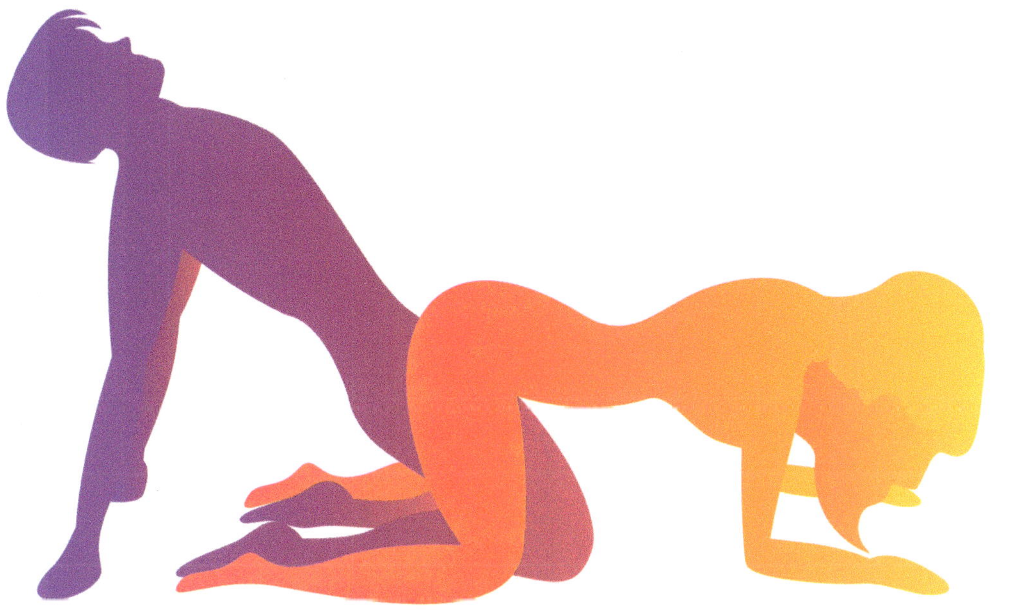

32

The Crouching Tiger:

The man is lying on the bed, legs hanging off the edge with his feet on the floor. The woman sits on him at the level of his pelvis, facing away. She places her legs on either side of his thighs and guides the penis into her vagina. She can lean on her partner's thighs or on the bed and rock back and forth.

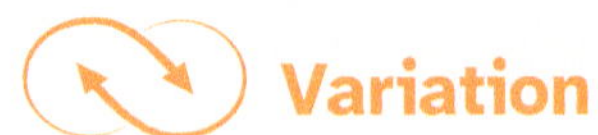

Variation

The man can slightly lift his torso by supporting himself on his forearms or hands. In this case, he can no longer touch or caress his partner. She dominates him entirely and can intensify the swinging motion by arching backward or leaning forward.

The Crouching Tiger

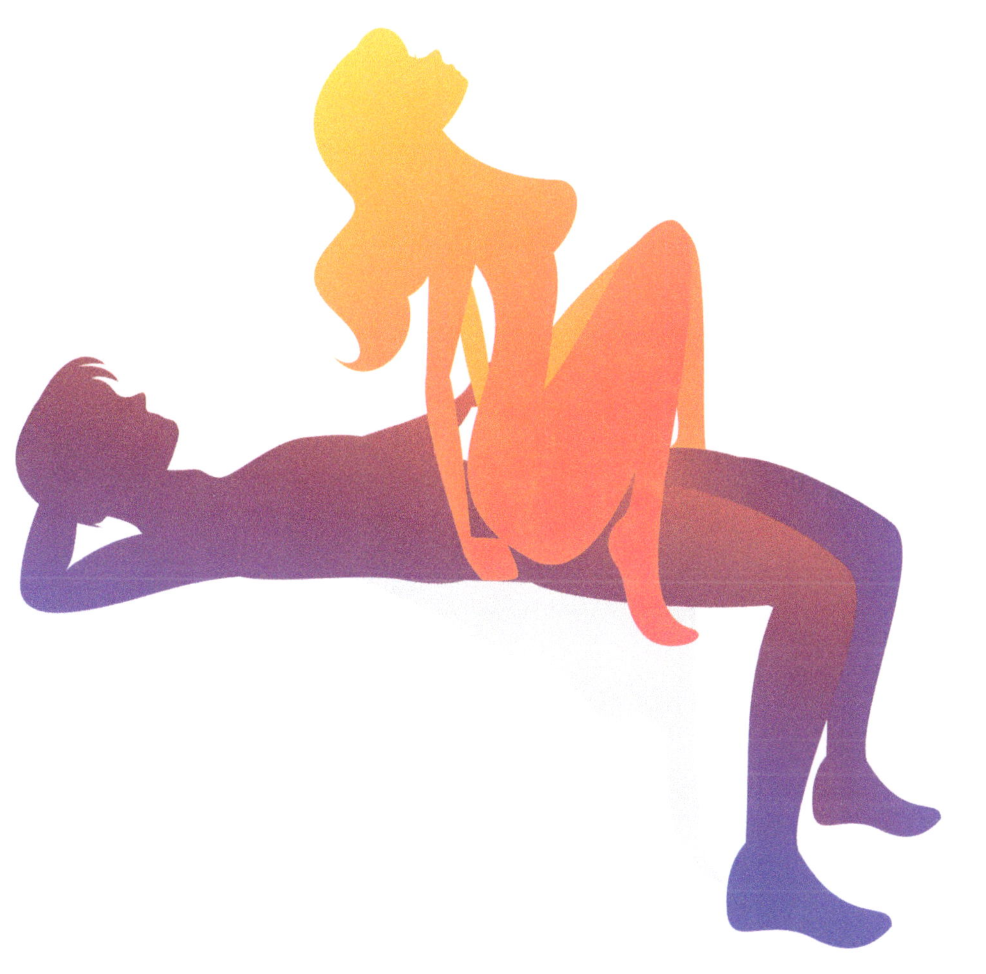

Splitting Bamboo:

The woman lies on her back. The man kneels in front of her so that they form a right angle. To achieve this, the woman's left leg rests on the bed between her partner's legs, while her right leg is placed on his shoulder.

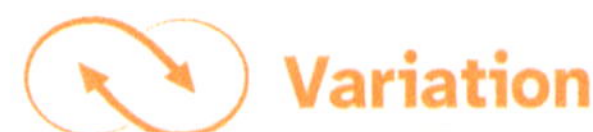 **Variation**

The woman can switch legs, placing it on her partner's opposite shoulder or adjusting the height by moving her pelvis. Each movement varies the penetration angle, offering enhanced sensations for both partners.

Splitting Bamboo

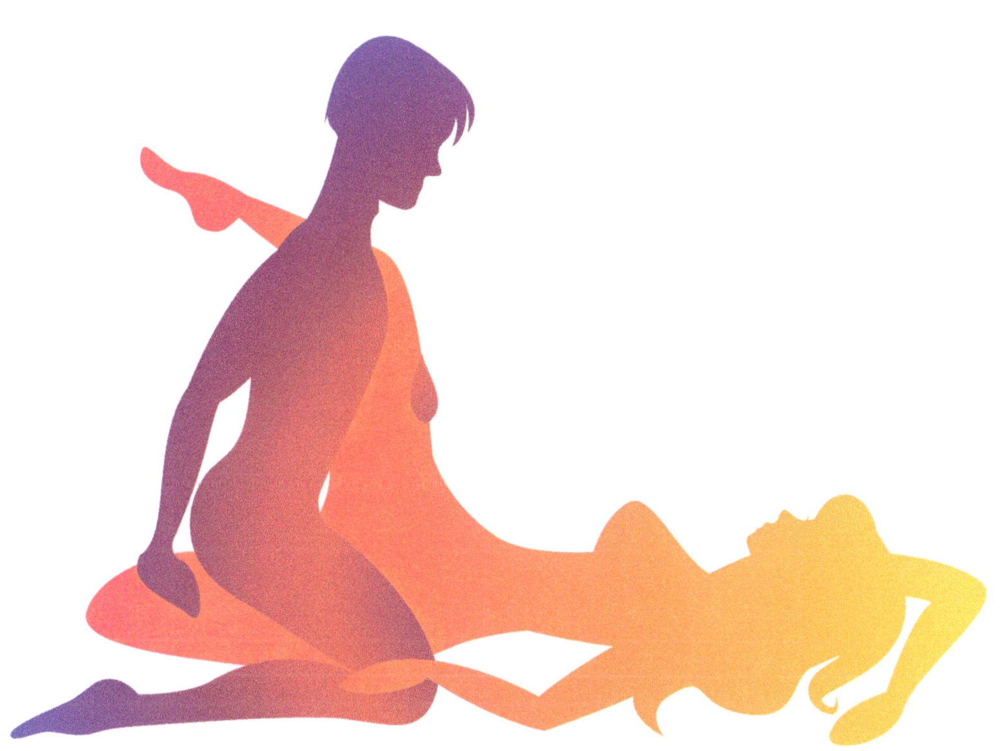

34

The Propeller:

The missionary position is the starting point. A few thrusts later, the man, without exiting his partner, performs a 180-degree rotation to end up facing her back and continues his pelvic movements. The woman positions her partner's legs under her arms and has her hands free to caress his buttocks.

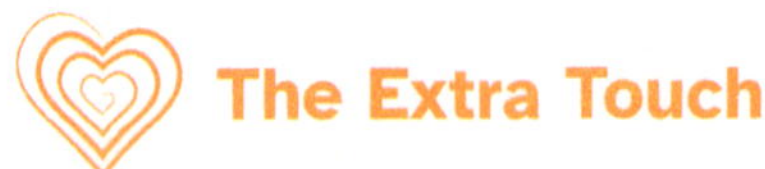

The Extra Touch

For a perfect rotation, the woman can place a small cushion under her pelvis to elevate it and have a more suitable angle for the maneuver.

The Propeller

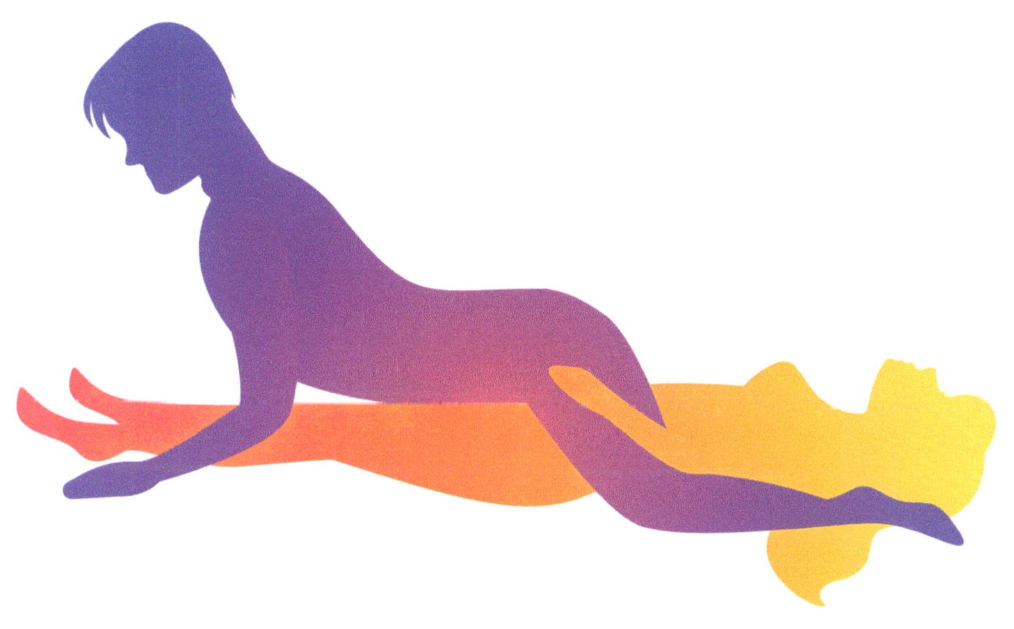

35

The Lotus Blossom:

The man sits on the floor, cross-legged. Once in position, the woman sits facing him on his lap, wrapping her legs around his waist.

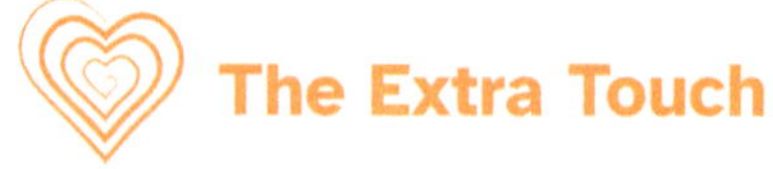

The Extra Touch

To maintain the cross-legged position more easily and relieve his back, the man can lean against a support, such as a wall.

The Lotus Blossom

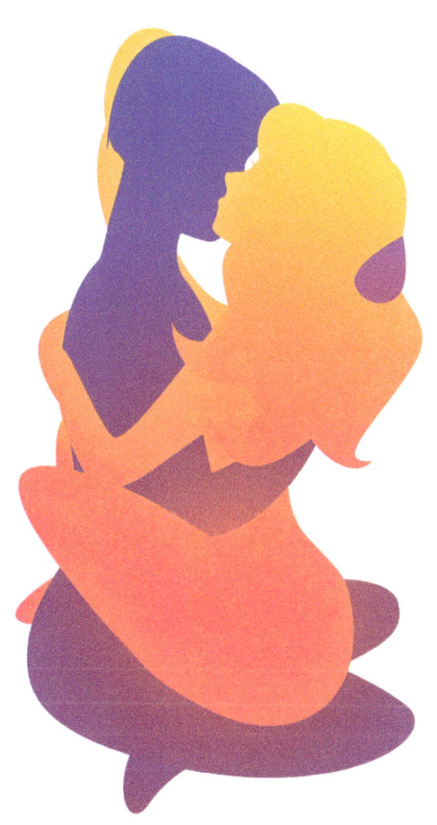

36

The Padlock:

The woman sits elevated on a piece of furniture (a table, a desk, a sink, a washing machine...) and leans backward, supporting herself with her hands. She wraps her legs around the man's hips, who stands facing her. He grips his partner's hips (or her buttocks, or the edges of the furniture...) to initiate a deep back-and-forth movement.

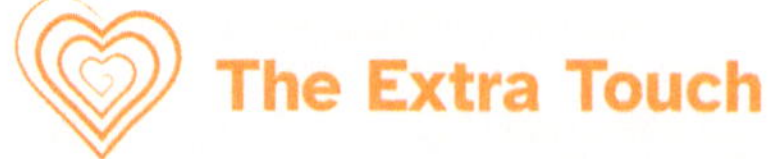 **The Extra Touch**

This position can be practiced anywhere, especially in unusual places! By arching slightly, the man ensures better penetration.

The Padlock

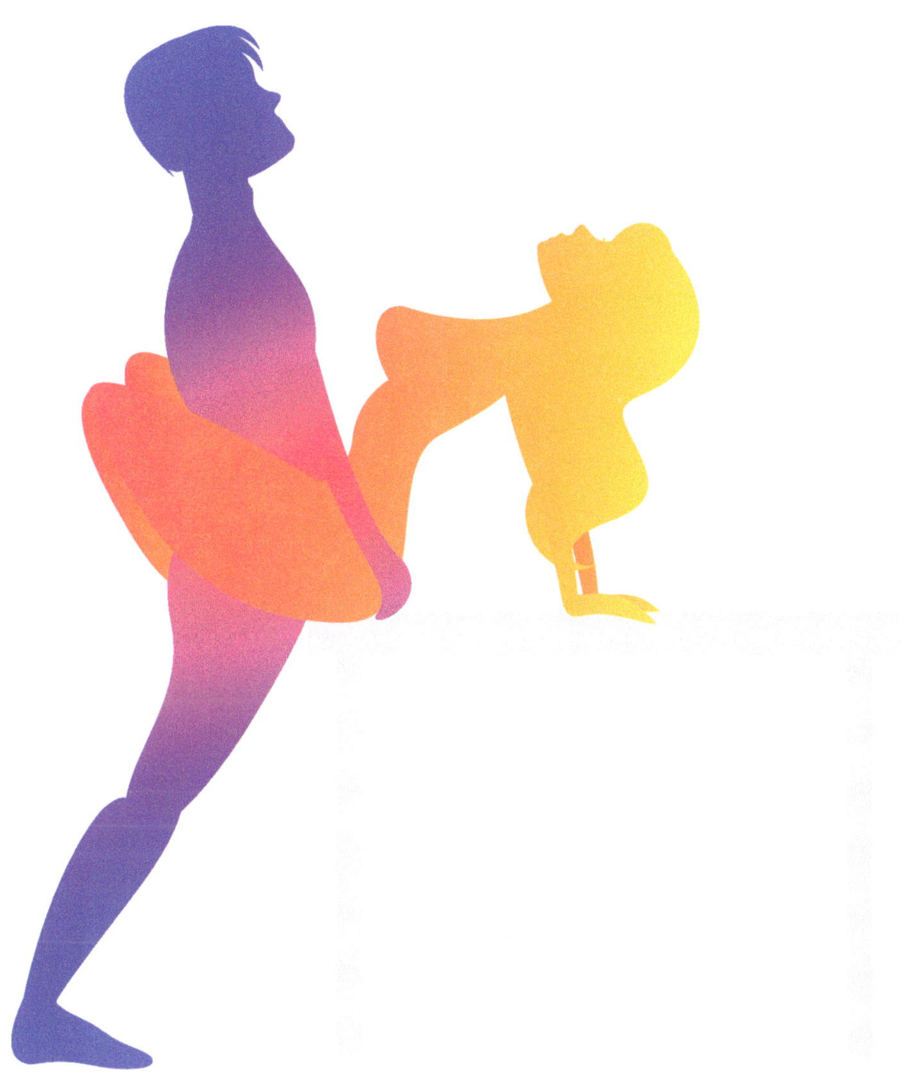

37

The Deckchair:

The woman lies on her back and raises her legs. The man sits facing her, with both legs on either side of his partner. He lifts his pelvis slightly to facilitate penetration and supports himself with his hands on the bed behind him. The woman rests her ankles on his shoulders.

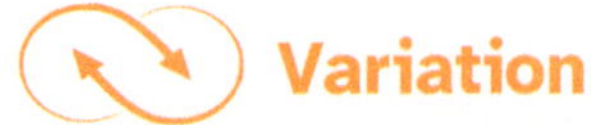 **Variation**

A less athletic variation involves staying on the forearms rather than the hands.

The Deckchair

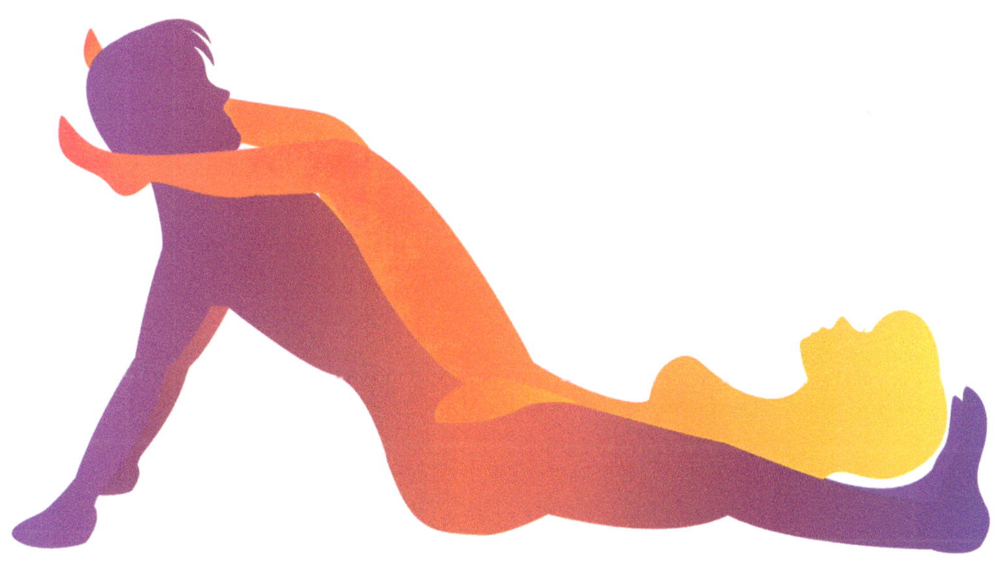

The Double Decker:

The man lies down, and the woman straddles him, facing away. Guiding her partner's sex inside her, she leans back on her forearms. Then, by moving her legs, she initiates vertical back-and-forth movements.

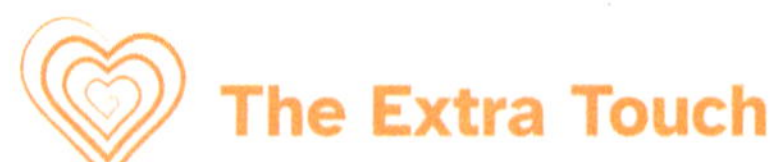

The Extra Touch

In this position, the man is quite passive, but he has free hands to caress his partner's breasts or clitoris.

The Double Decker

The Candle:

The woman lies on her back and spreads her legs. The man kneels in front of her. He lifts her legs and holds her in this position by gripping her ankles or thighs.

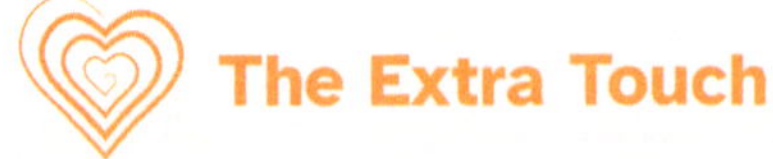 **The Extra Touch**

To stimulate his partner's clitoris, the man can open and close her legs, mimicking wing flaps.

The Candle

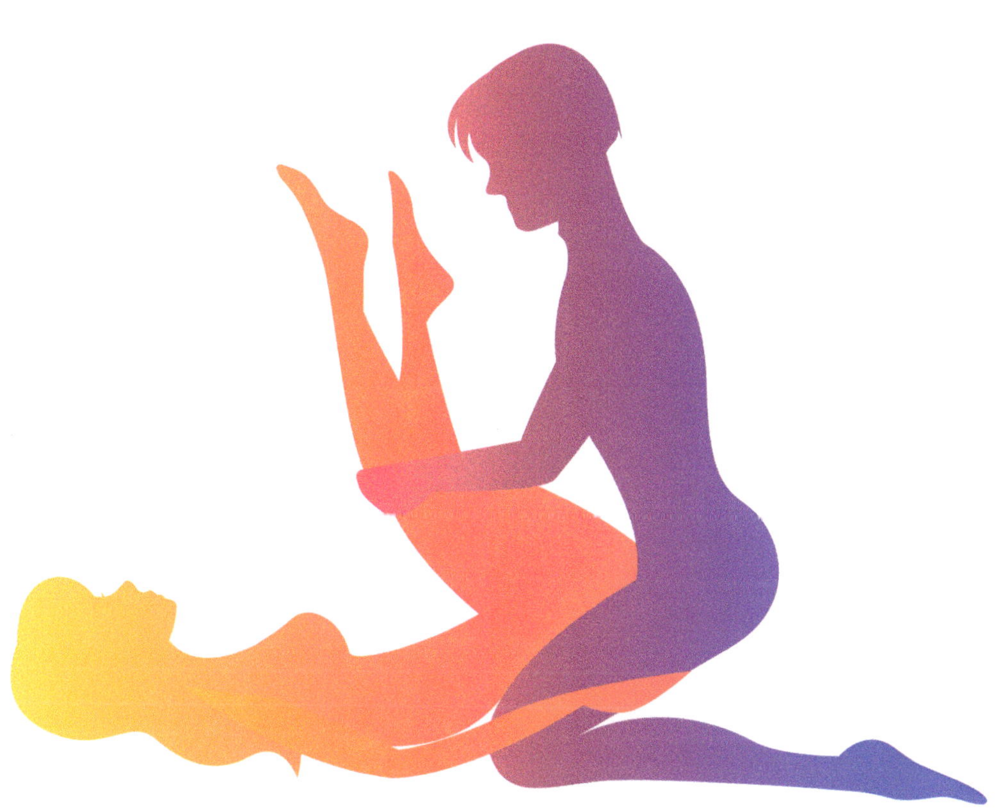

The Spider:

The man is seated, slightly leaning back and supported by his hands. His legs are extended and slightly apart. The woman straddles him. She also leans slightly back and supports herself on the floor or mattress with her hands. Her legs are on either side of her partner, with her knees at his shoulders.

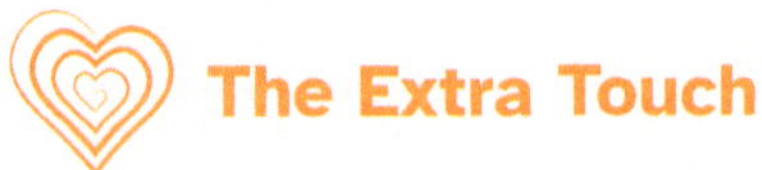

The Extra Touch

In this position, the woman takes the lead. She can arch more or less, squeeze her thighs or not, and move at her desired pace. She offers the man an exciting view of her sex.

The Spider

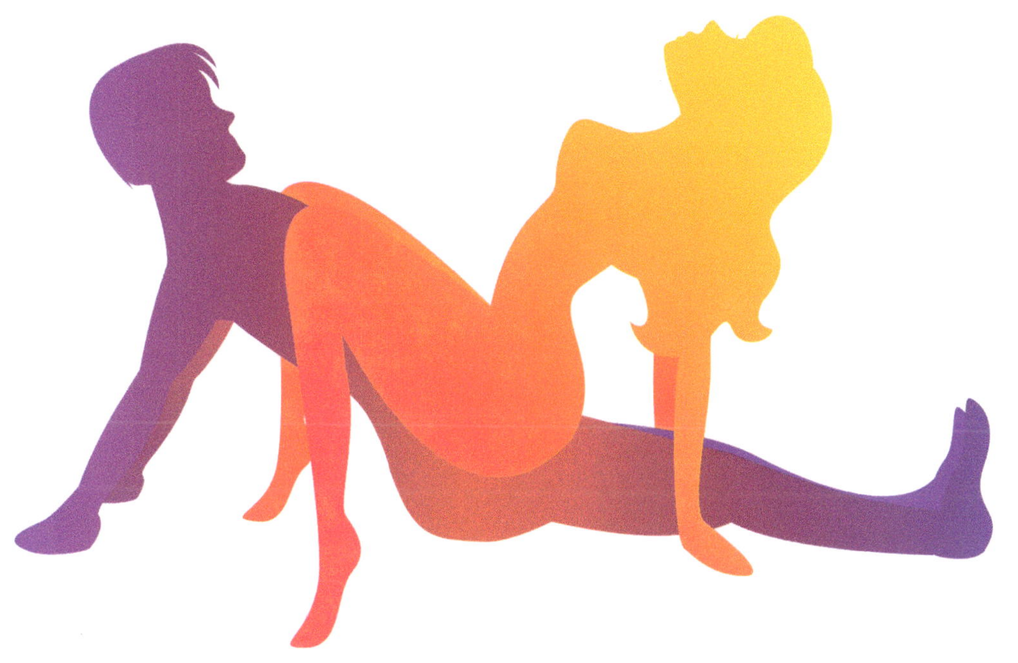

41

The Star:

The woman lies on her back with her head resting on a pillow. She stretches one leg and bends the other, knee toward the ceiling. The man sits astride her outstretched leg, tilting his torso backward and supporting himself with his hands.

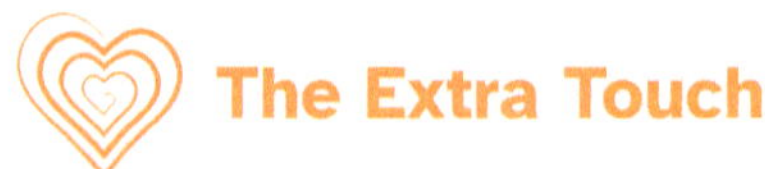 **The Extra Touch**

In this position, the man controls penetration, and the woman can completely let go. It's ideal between two more acrobatic positions or for a sensual cuddling session.

The Star

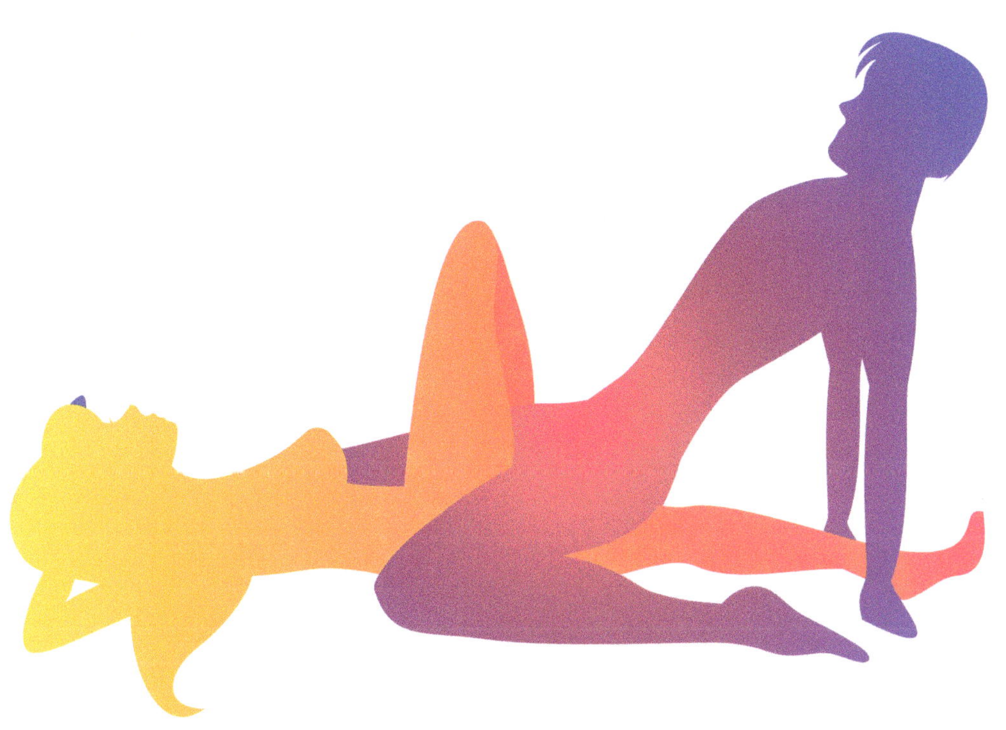

From Behind:

Both partners are standing. The woman turns her back to the man and slightly leans forward. The man positions himself behind her and grasps her hips. For more stability, the woman can lean against a wall or grip her lover's buttocks. If her partner is much taller, she can wear heels or stand on a support to ease penetration.

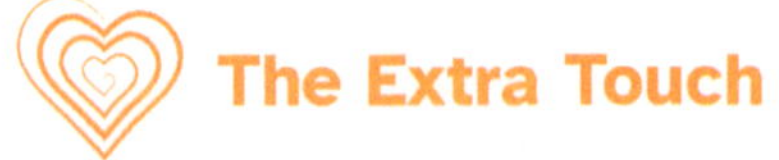 **The Extra Touch**

The man can also lean forward to kiss his partner's back or neck or whisper naughty words in her ear.

From Behind

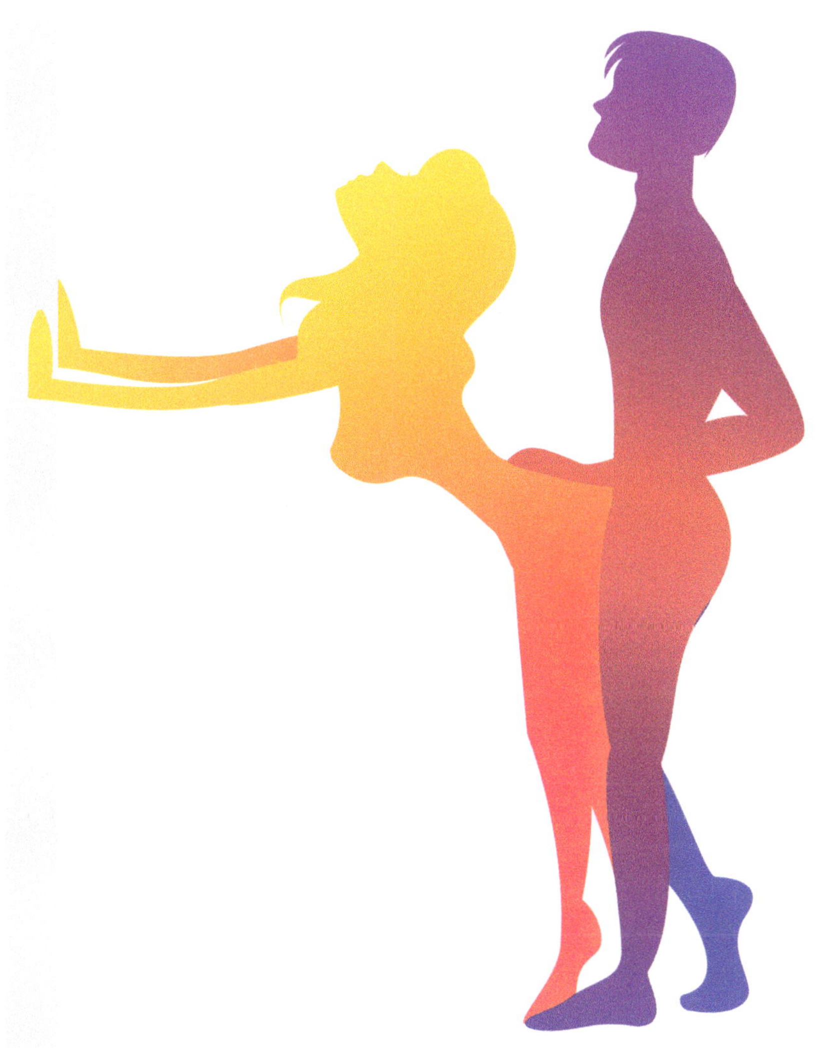

43

The Crisscross:

The woman lies on her side, her back to her partner. The man places himself perpendicular to her, between her thighs, and penetrates her while leaning on her shoulders.

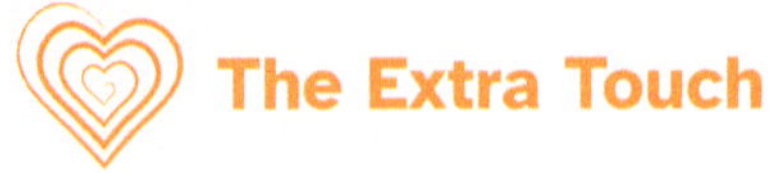 **The Extra Touch**

This position is a variation of doggy style and is particularly effective for the pleasure of both partners. The man can perform deep thrusts while being held snugly by the pressure of the woman's thighs.

The Crisscross

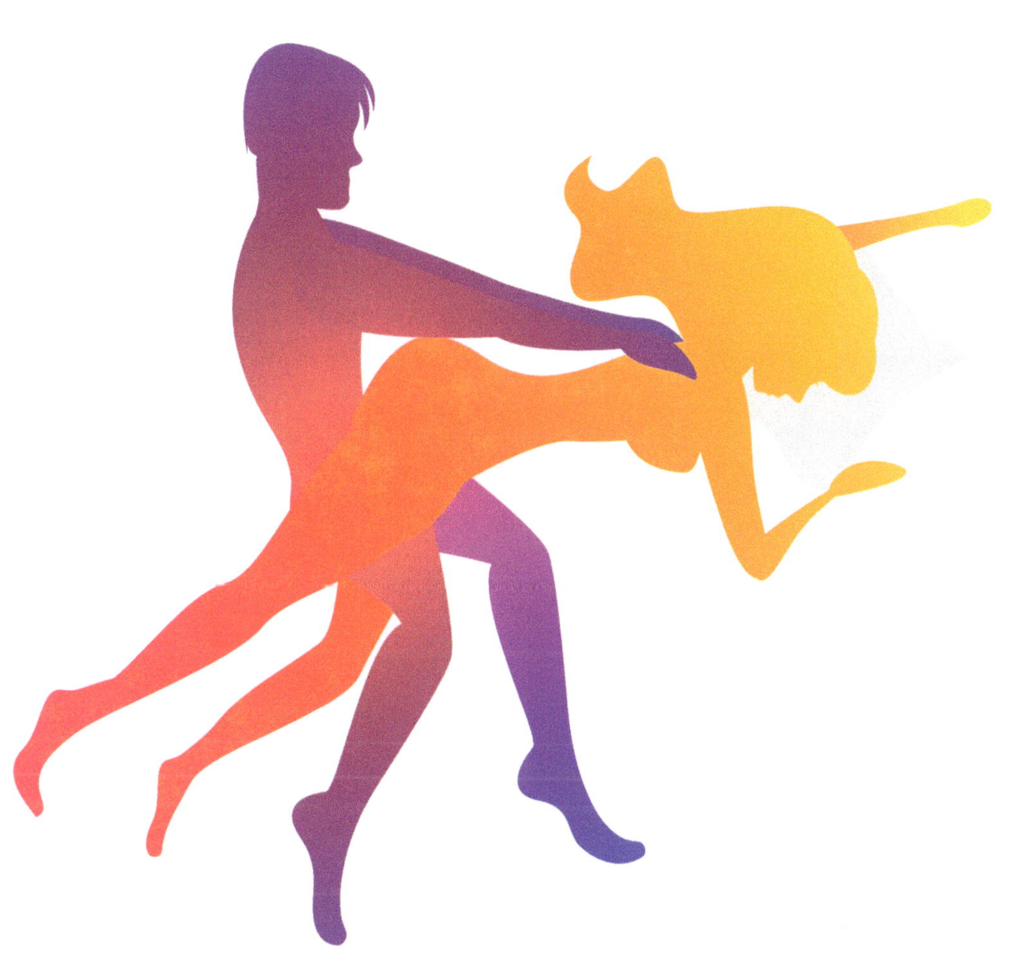

44

The Prone Tiger:

The man sits with his legs extended. The woman lies flat on her stomach on her partner's legs, pelvis to pelvis, so their sexes are at the same level. Penetration is gentle but deep. By supporting herself on her forearms, the woman creates an up-and-down motion.

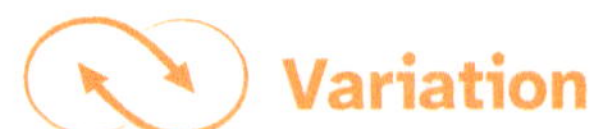 **Variation**

The man can lean back and lie on his back. The partners then explore the position of the Grand X, offering a different penetration angle.

The Prone Tiger

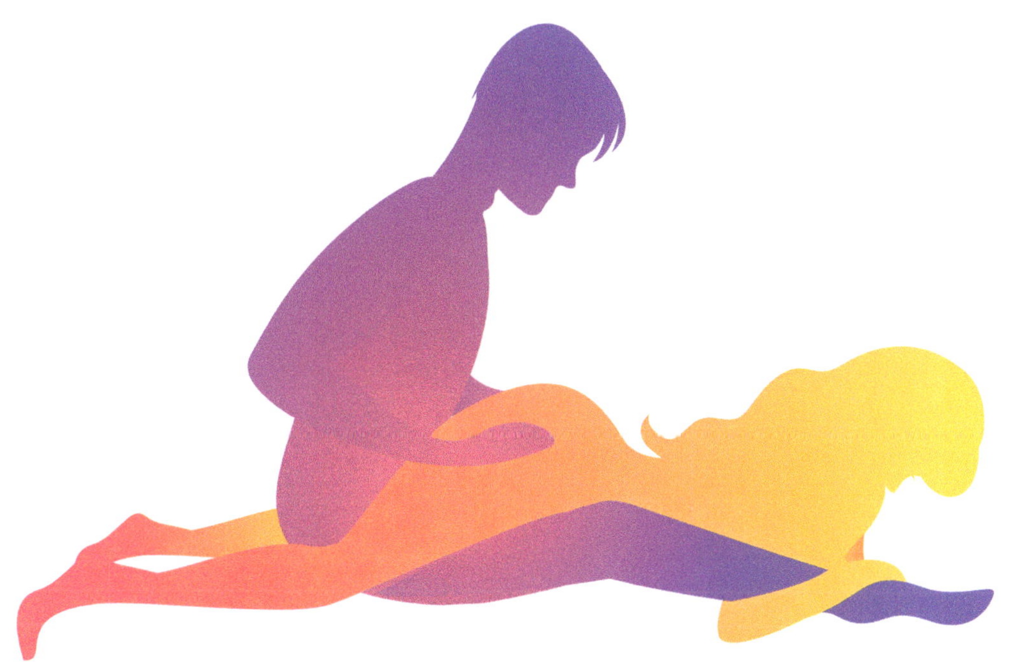

45

The Lap Top:

The man is seated on a chair, armchair, or sofa. The woman straddles him, places her hands around his neck, and lifts her legs to put them on his shoulders. Her partner firmly grips her hips and pushes them forward and backward to accelerate or slow down the movements.

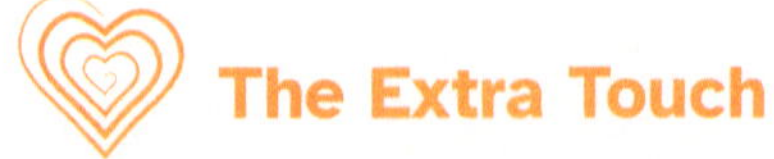

The Extra Touch

To facilitate penetration and set the pace, the woman can push her feet against the chair's backrest.

The Lap Top

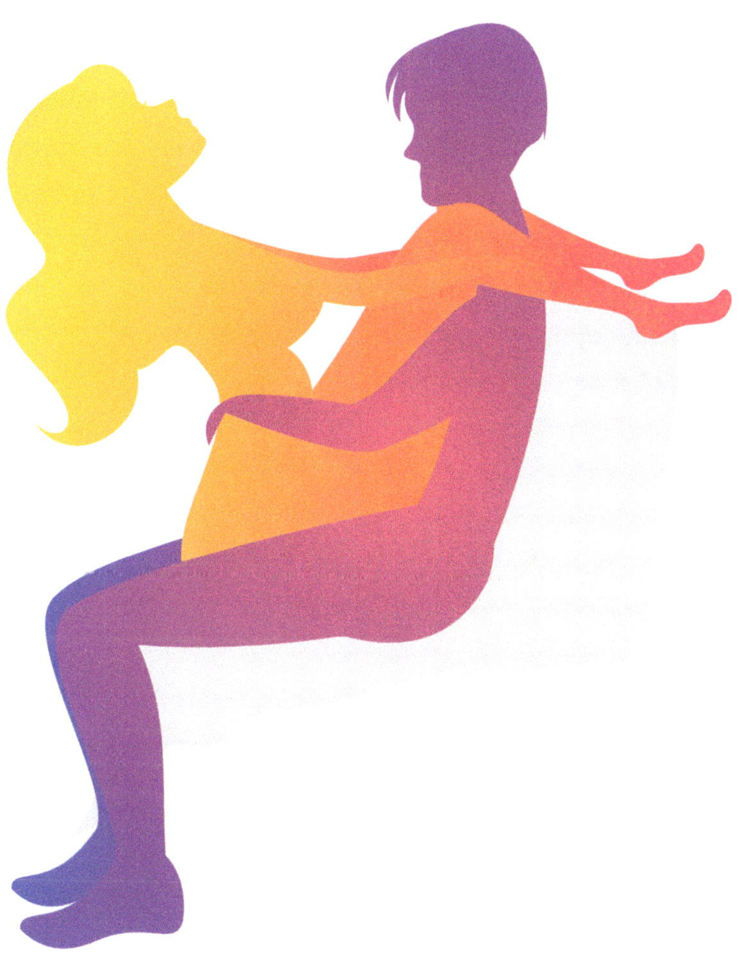

46

The Snail:

The woman lies on her back. The man slides between her thighs, on his knees. He grabs his partner's ankles and places them on his shoulders. Penetration is even deeper if the man leans forward and lifts his partner's pelvis.

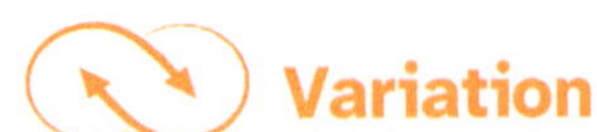 **Variation**

Instead of placing both feet on his partner's shoulders, the woman leaves one leg extended on the mattress or the floor.

The Snail

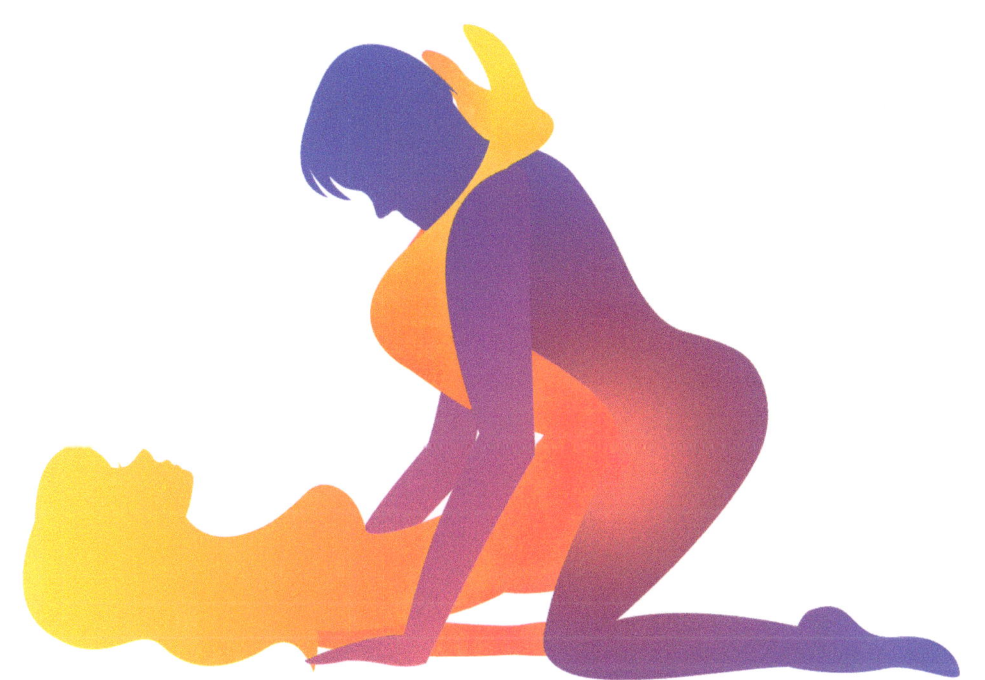

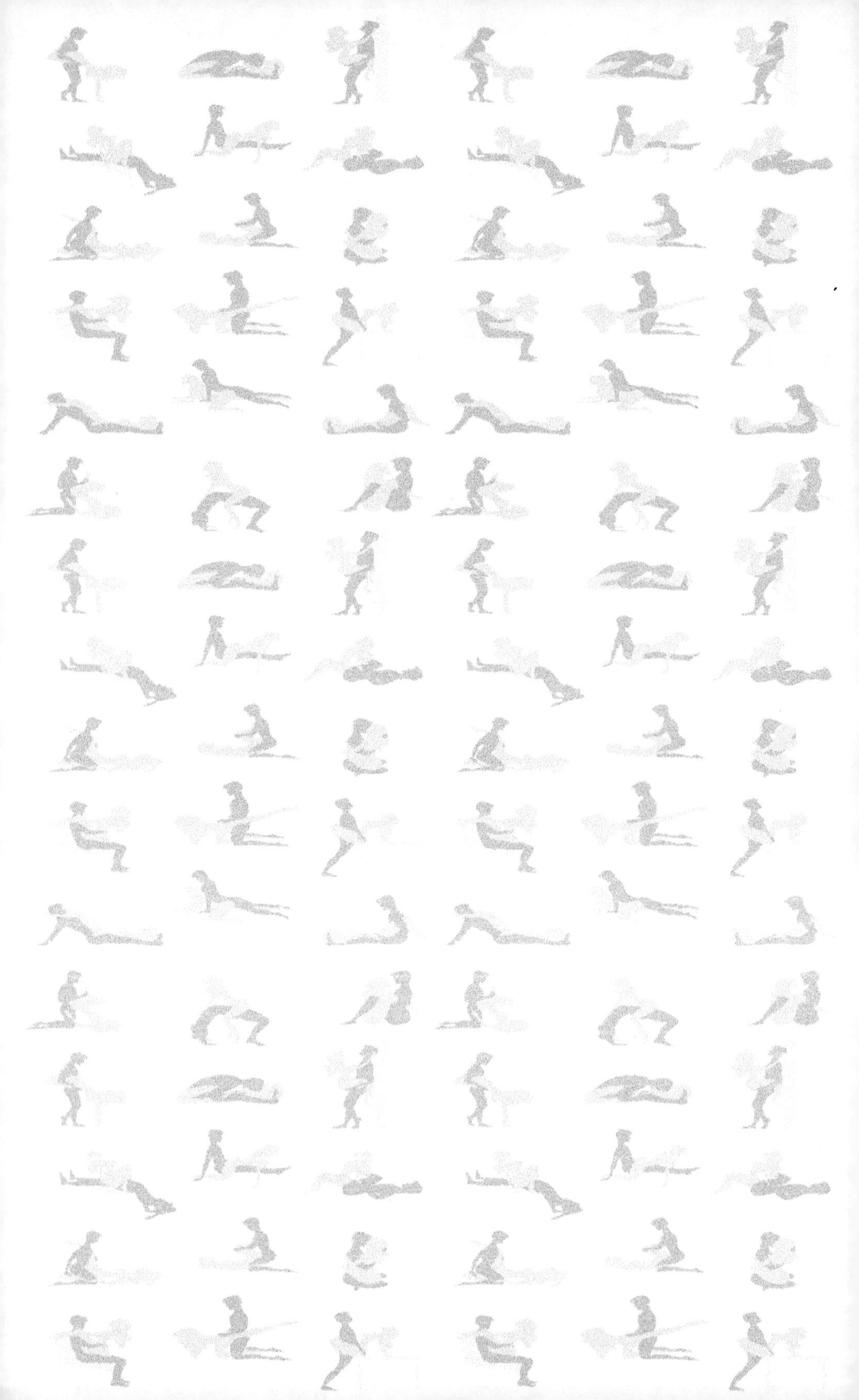

Enchanting Acrobatics

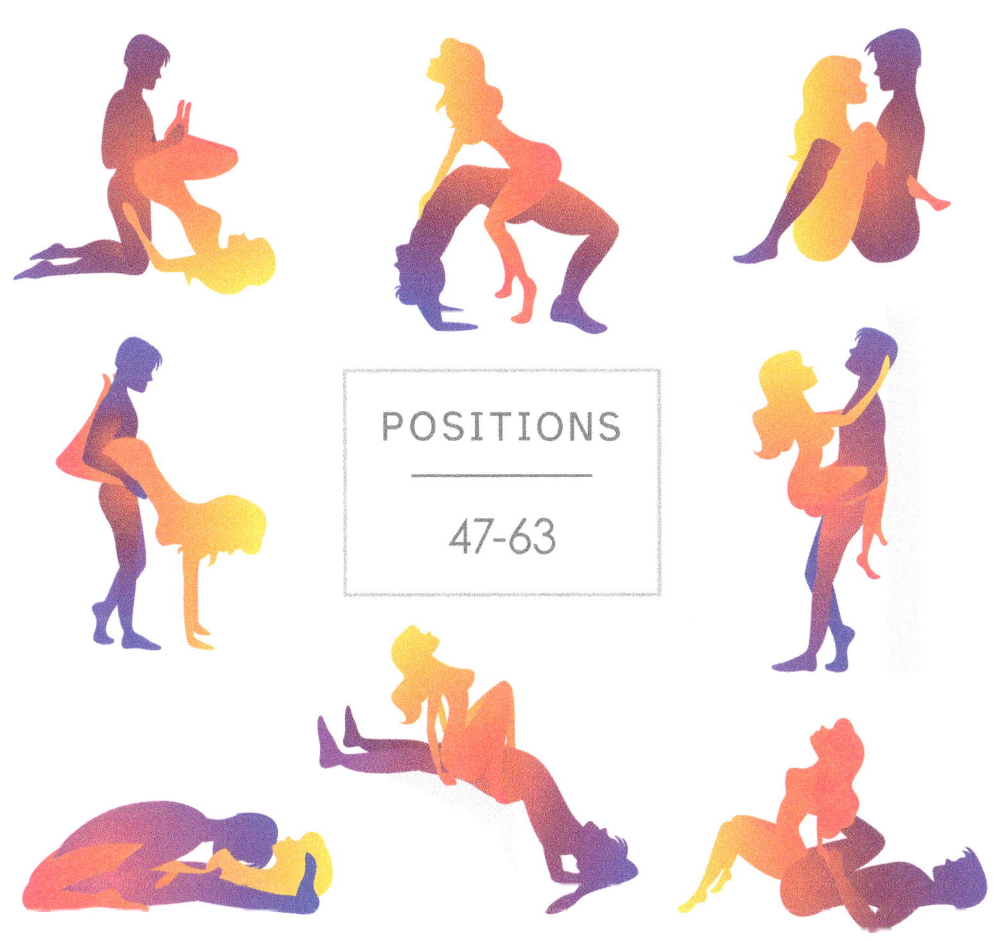

47

The Bridge:

The man assumes the bridge position, legs bent, supported by his arms, with his abdomen facing the sky. The woman delicately straddles him, fitting onto his pelvis, and performs gentle hip rotations.

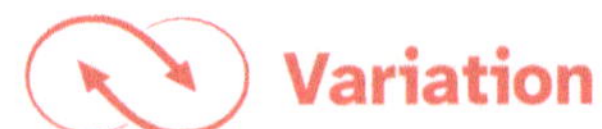 **Variation**

To vary the sensations, the woman can either face her partner or turn her back to him. The man, in turn, can place his back on a flat surface at a suitable height or on a mound of cushions for a more comfortable ride.

The Bridge

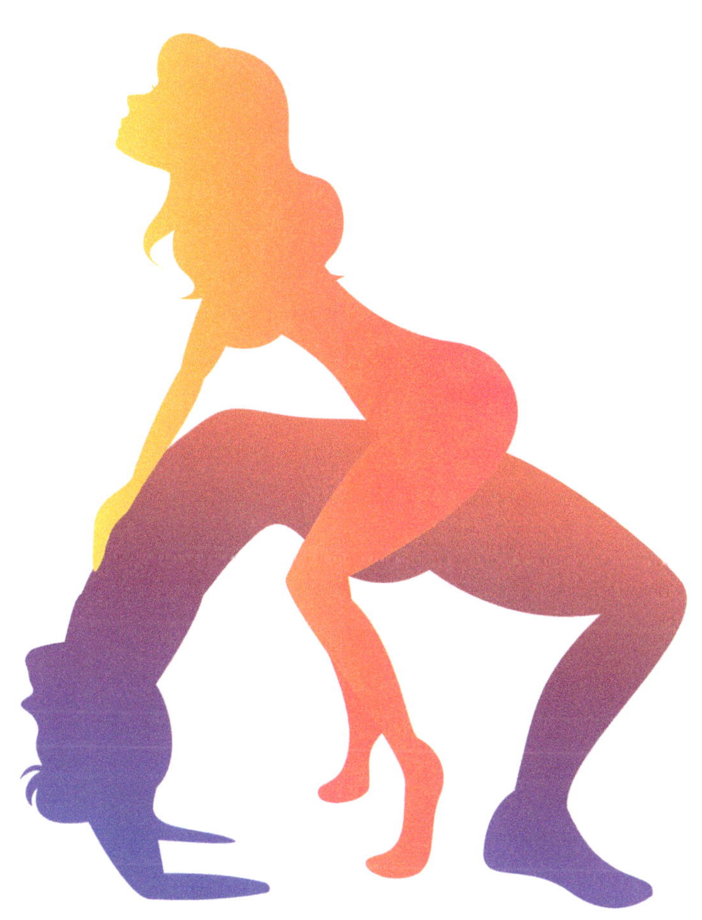

48

The Backward Slide:

The man sits on the bed or on a chair. The woman straddles him, positioning her legs on either side of his body and leaning backward while supporting herself with her hands on the floor. The man then initiates a back-and-forth motion.

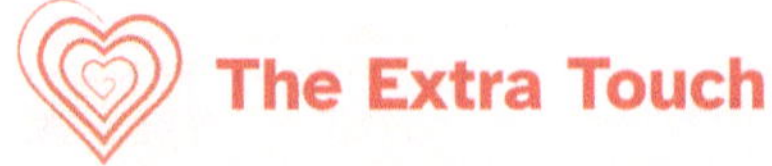 **The Extra Touch**

The man has free hands to stimulate highly erogenous areas of the woman, such as her breasts and clitoris.

The Backward Slide

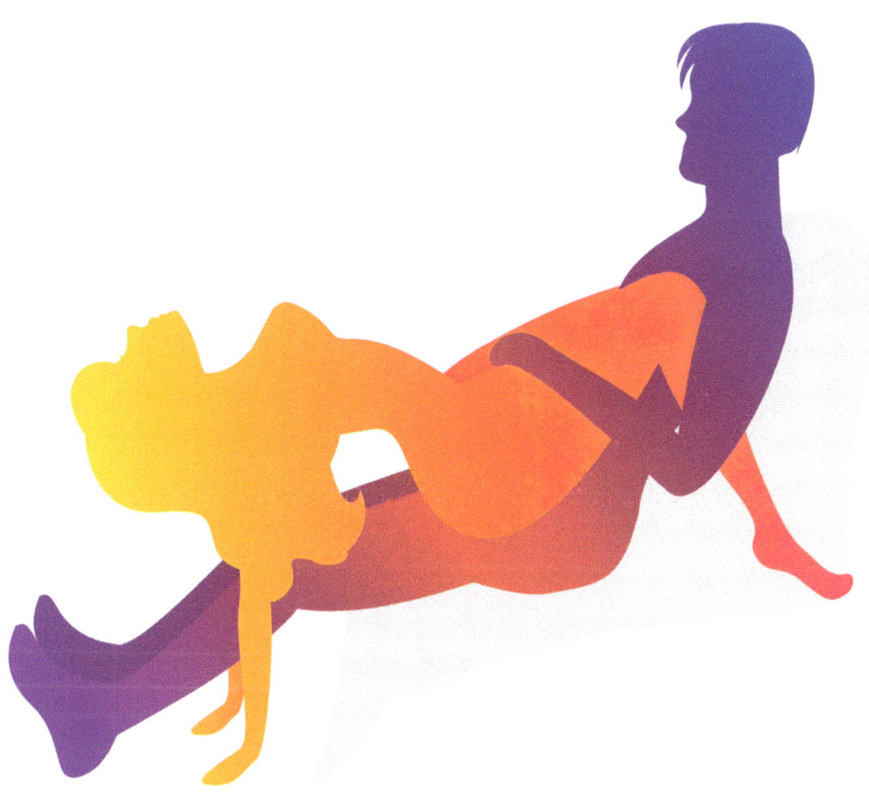

49

The Plough:

The woman positions herself at the edge of the bed or a sofa, facing the floor, with her elbows supporting her. The man, standing behind her, lifts her legs to the height of her pelvis. While holding his partner's thighs on either side of his pelvis, he penetrates her at his own pace.

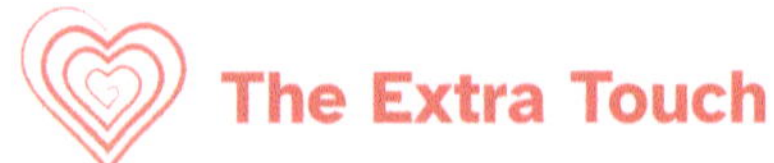 **The Extra Touch**

A more athletic variation of doggy style that offers a different angle of penetration.

The Plough

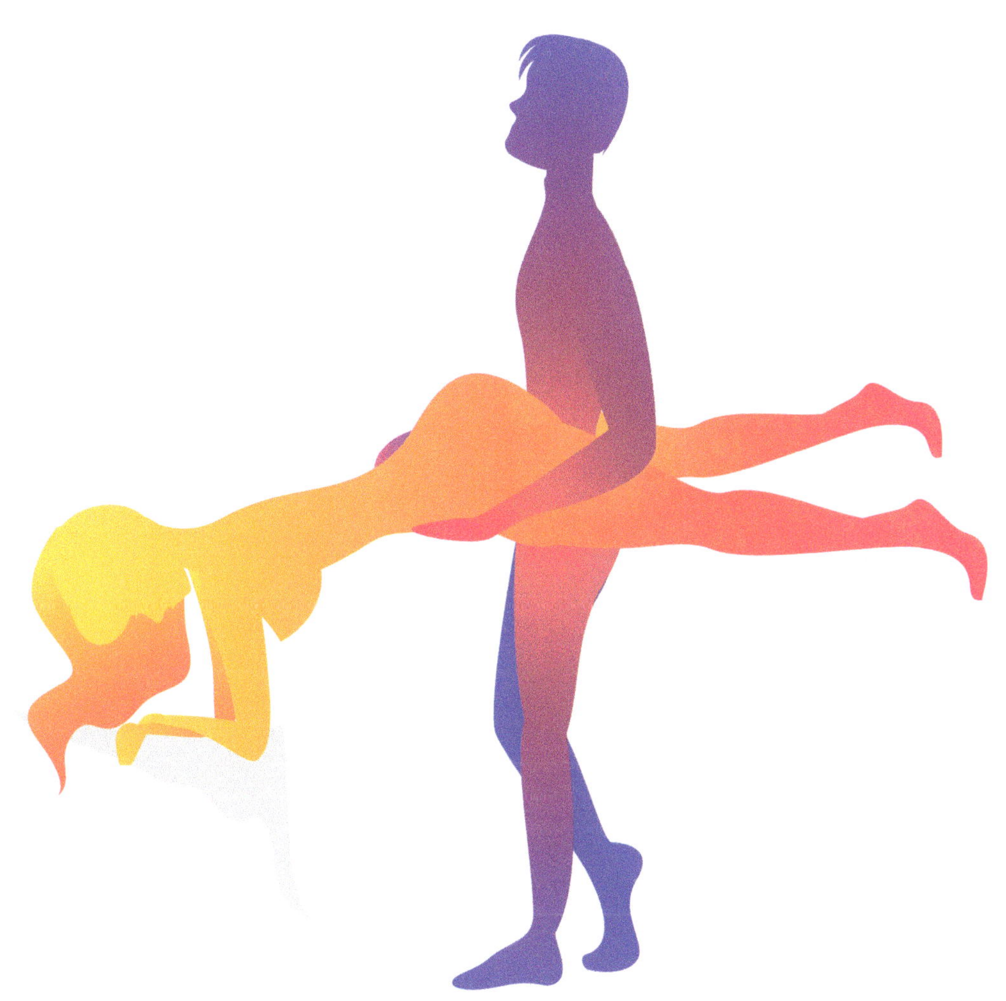

The Challenge:

The woman stands on a stool or a chair and bends her knees to position her buttocks backward. To maintain balance, she places her hands and forearms on her knees and thighs. The man stands behind her, holding her hips or buttocks and initiating a back-and-forth motion.

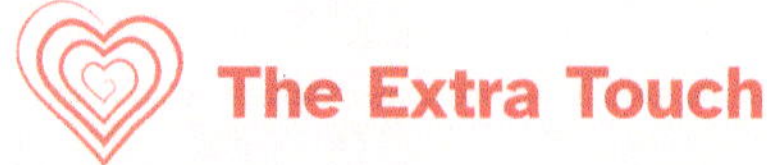

The Extra Touch

To make the position more comfortable, place the stool or chair in front of a high piece of furniture for the woman to lean against.

The Challenge

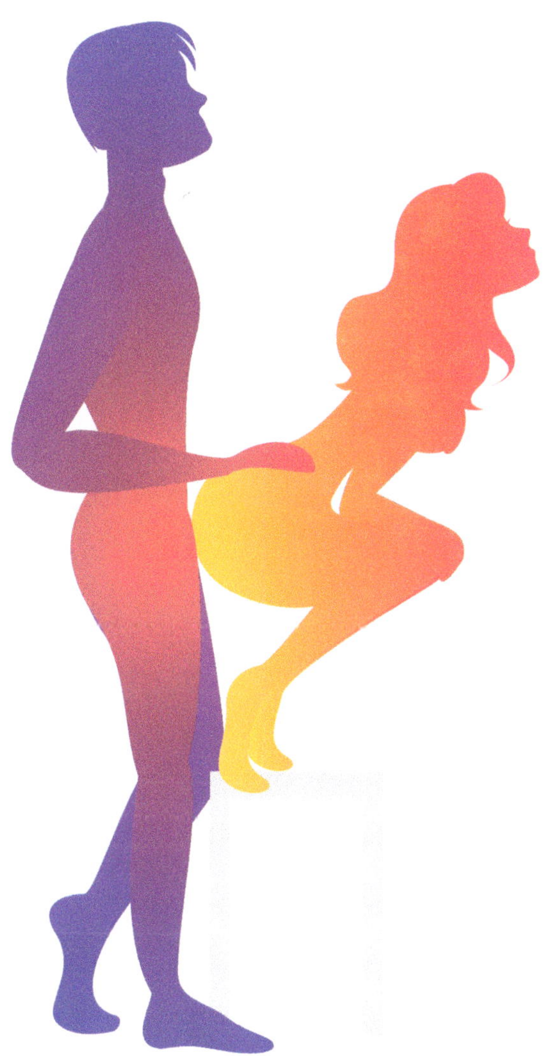

The Dolphin:

The woman lies on her back, then lifts her hips while keeping her feet, shoulders, and head on the floor. The man kneels between her legs and lifts her while holding her pelvis with his hands on her buttocks.

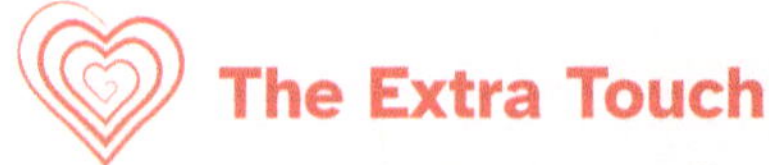

The Extra Touch

If the position seems too acrobatic, place a large cushion under the woman's back to make the posture more accessible and comfortable.

The Dolphin

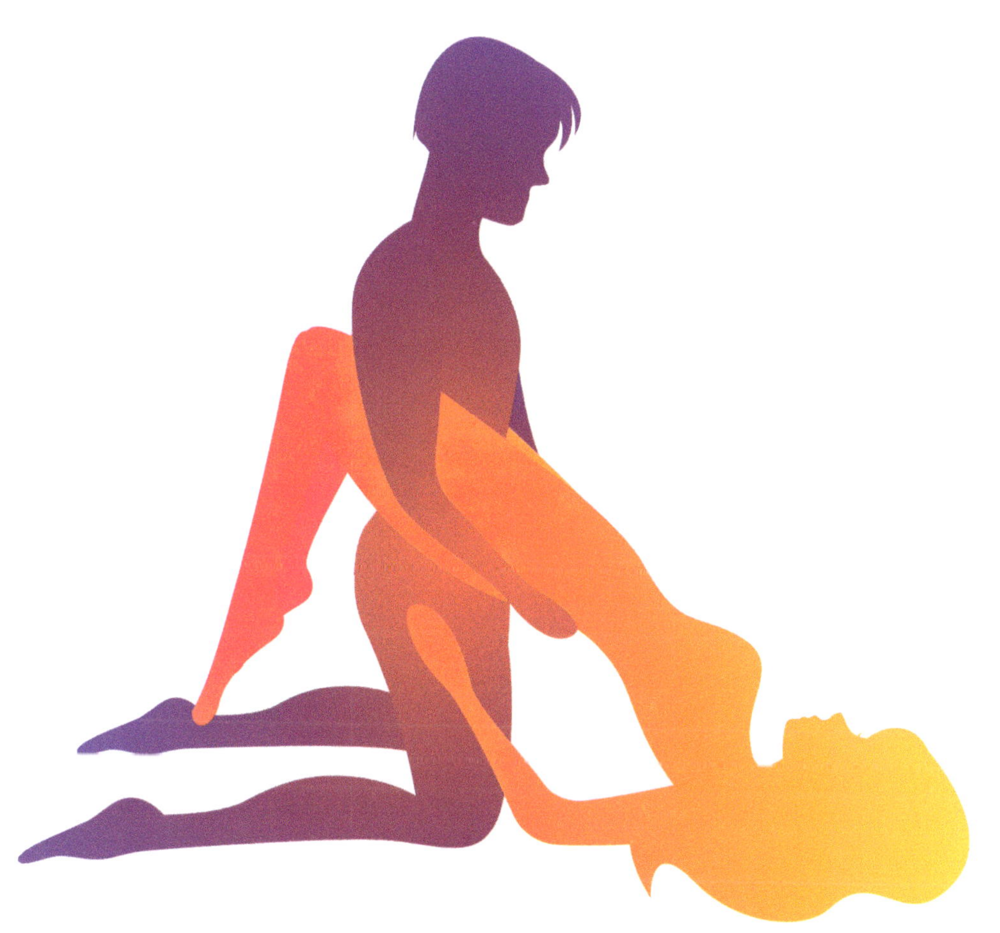

The Erotic V:

The woman sits at the edge of a table and raises her legs to place them on the man's shoulders, who stands facing her. To maintain balance, she grips her partner's shoulders or supports herself behind by placing her hands on the table. The man, in turn, holds her by the hips and ensures deep back-and-forth movements.

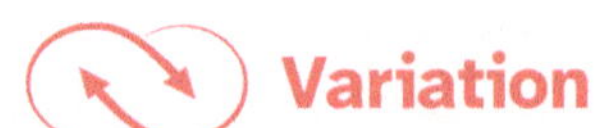

Variation

Sensations are heightened if the woman crosses her legs behind her partner's neck!

The Erotic V

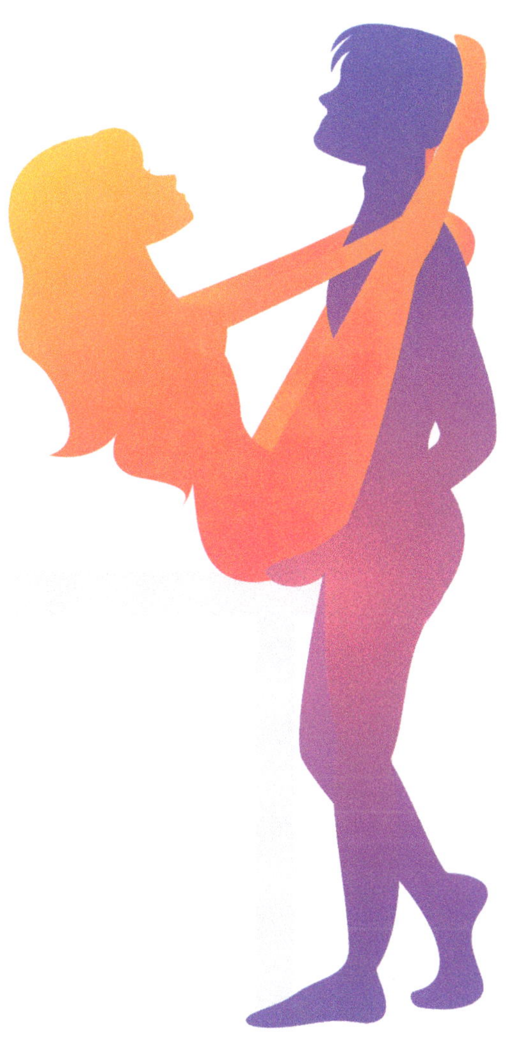

53

The Rowing Boat:

The partners sit face to face, locking eyes. They spread their legs and move as close to each other as possible until their sexes touch. Once in position, they lift their legs. For better stability, they hold each other by the ankles.

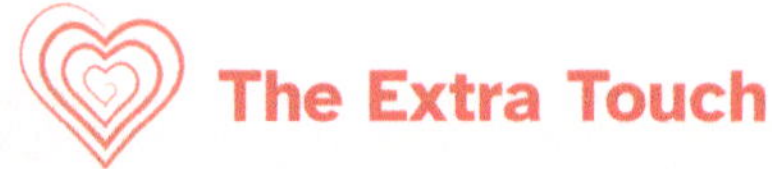 **The Extra Touch**

One of the most challenging positions in the Kamasutra, requiring skill and a degree of flexibility, but offering intense orgasms due to an unusual penetration angle.

The Rowing Boat

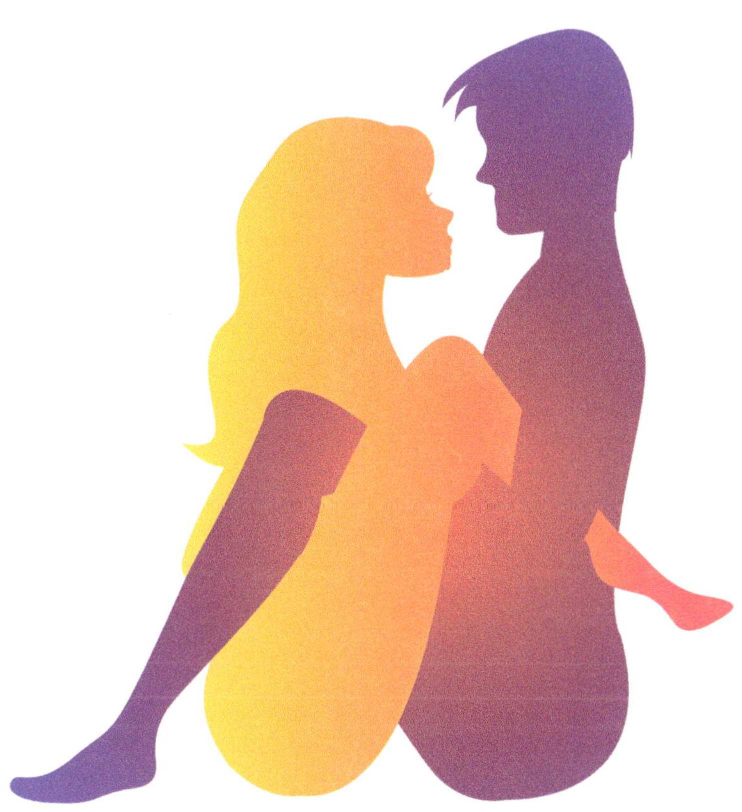

The Standing Wheelbarrow:

The woman kneels, forearms resting on a cushion. The man stands behind her, grasps her ankles, and positions them at the level of his pelvis. He adjusts the height by bending his legs more or less and initiates a back-and-forth motion.

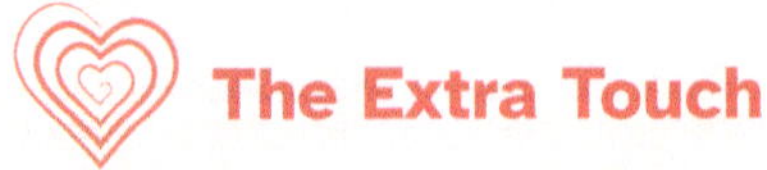 **The Extra Touch**

If there is a significant height difference between the partners, the woman can elevate herself by placing her forearms on a bench, a chair, or the edge of the mattress.

The Standing Wheelbarrow

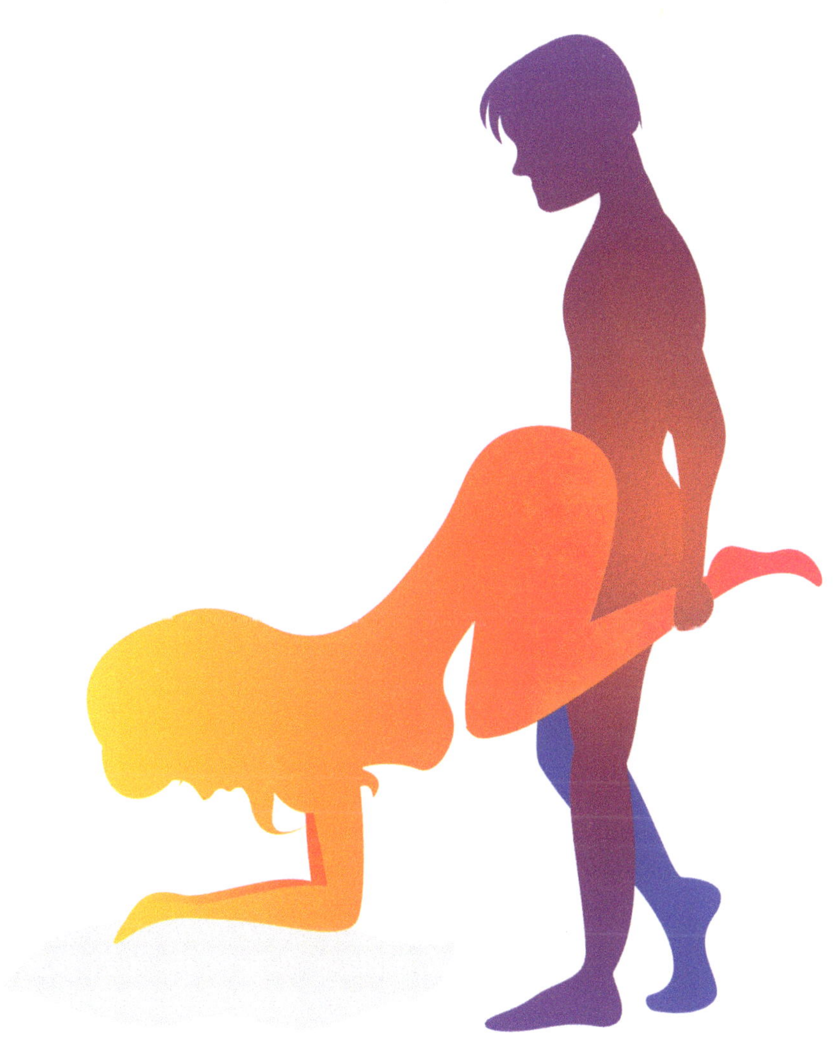

55

The Waterfall:

The man sits on a chair with his legs slightly apart. His partner sits on him, facing him and leaning backward. The man penetrates her and initiates a back-and-forth motion.

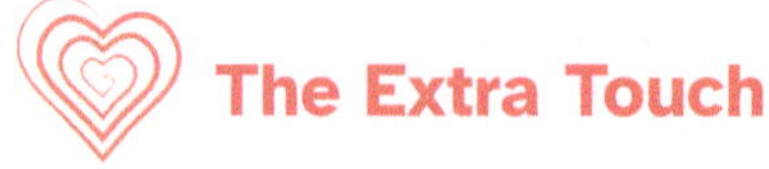

The Extra Touch

To increase his partner's excitement, the man can caress her breasts and clitoris.

The Waterfall

130

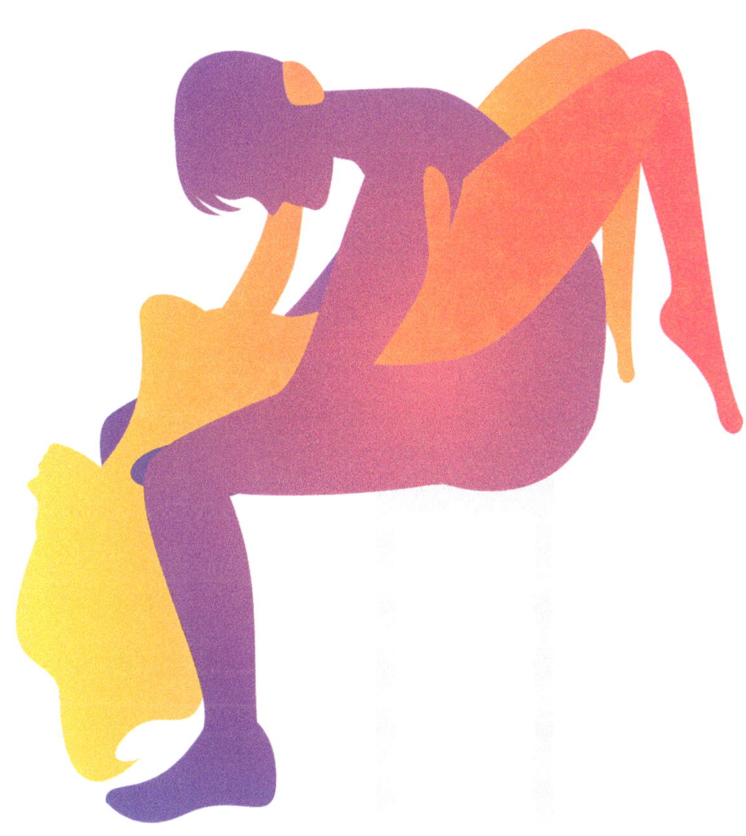

56

The Ape:

The man lies on his back and bends his knees toward his chest. The woman sits on him, facing away, using his feet as a "backrest." For added stability, she can hold onto her partner's hands. The rhythm of penetration is controlled by the man, who, by moving his feet, lifts his partner, creating an up-and-down motion.

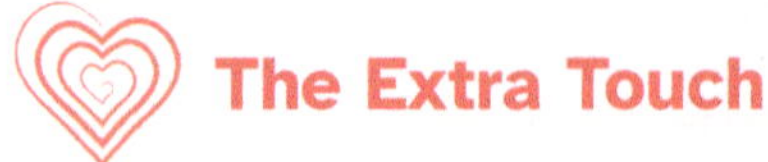 **The Extra Touch**

A position that requires leg strength from the man to lift his partner with each thrust. The woman should make herself as light as possible by engaging her thigh muscles to ease the effort.

The Ape

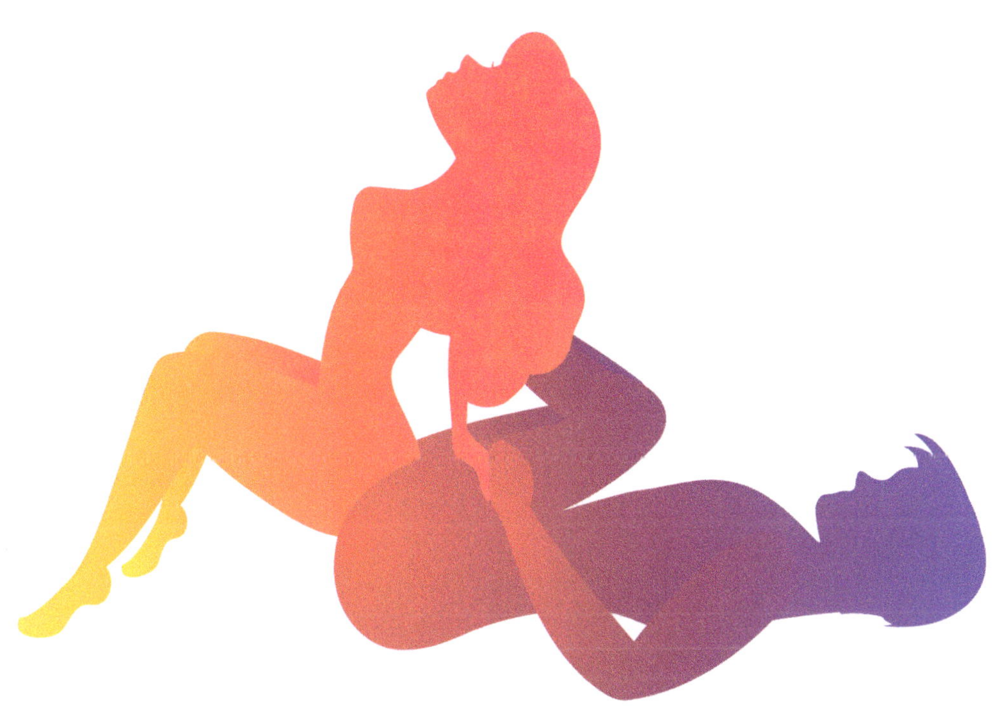

57

The Suspended Scissors:

The woman lies on her left side, legs scissored (left leg behind, right leg in front). The man stands with one foot on either side of her left thigh. In this position, he grasps her waist and right thigh, lifting her perpendicular to him. The woman supports herself on the floor with her left arm.

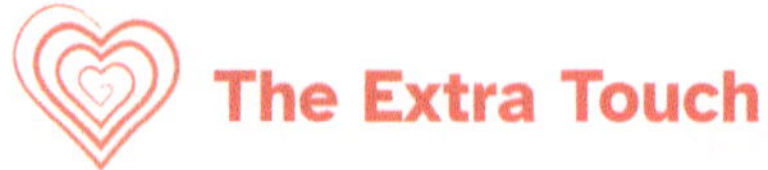 **The Extra Touch**

This position requires strong arms from both partners. To reduce the effort, the woman can place her left calf and foot on the edge of the bed.

The Suspended Scissors

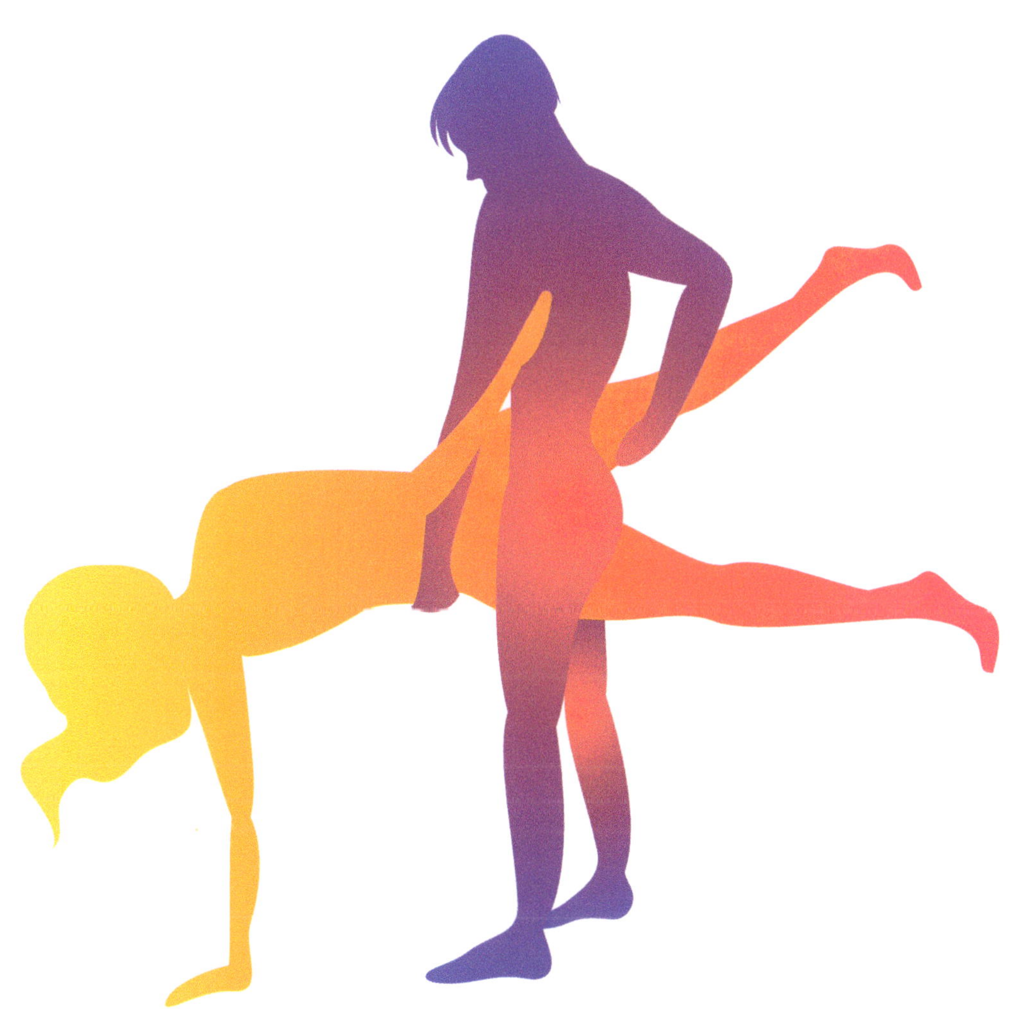

The Squat Balance:

The woman stands on the edge of a bed, a chair, or a low piece of furniture. The man stands behind her. The woman bends her knees to press her back against her partner's chest. The man places his hands under her buttocks to help her maintain this seated posture while she supports the back-and-forth movement with her forearms.

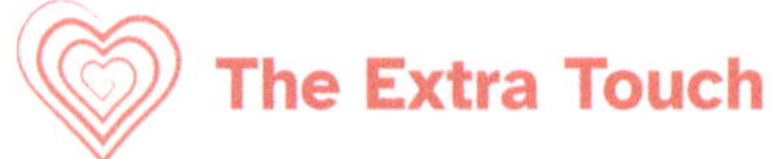 **The Extra Touch**

To maintain balance, the woman can lean her upper body slightly forward.

The Squat Balance

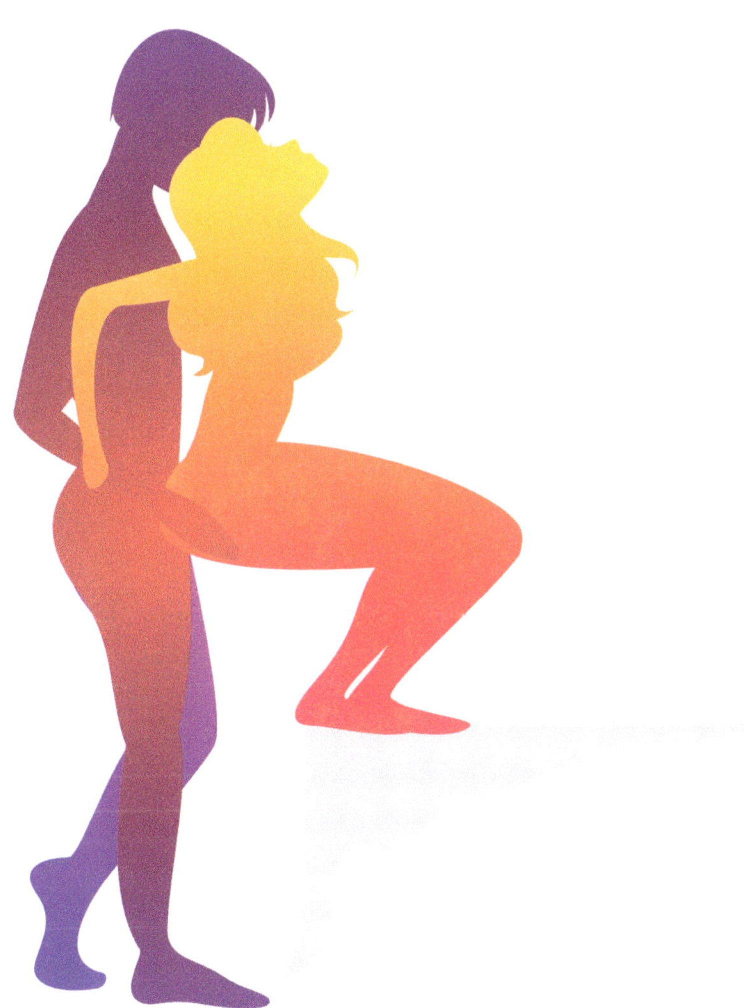

The Shoulder Stand:

The woman lies down, and the man kneels in front of her. He raises her legs vertically so that her back no longer touches the bed. She supports herself only on her shoulder blades, neck, and head. For added comfort and balance, the woman can hold onto her partner's thighs. Her ankles rest on her partner's shoulders, serving as support to keep her pelvis elevated. The man supports her by holding her buttocks.

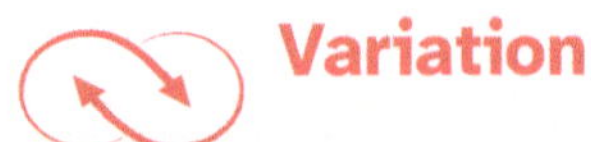 **Variation**

The position is the same as the The Shoulder Stand, but instead of placing her ankles on the man's shoulders, the woman positions her thighs on either side of her partner's chest.

The Shoulder Stand

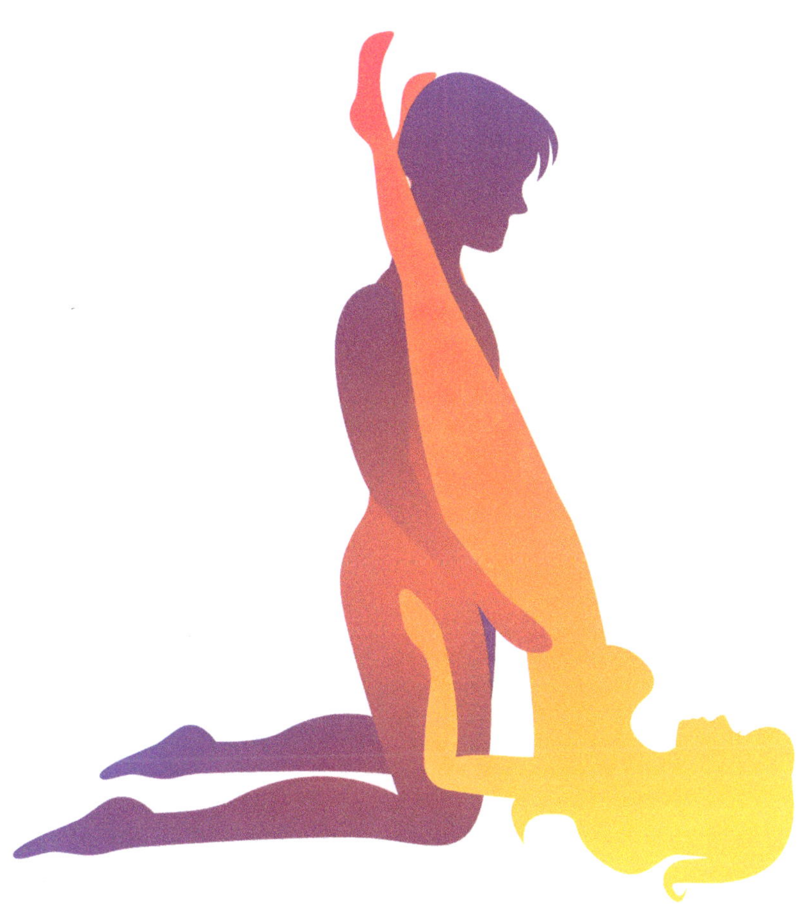

The Supernova:

The man lies on his back at the edge of the bed, with his upper body outside the bed. His head rests on the floor or on a pillow for greater comfort. The woman sits on him at the level of his lower abdomen, folding her legs and placing her feet on either side of her partner's buttocks. She leans slightly backward and places her hands flat behind her. She takes charge and sets the rhythm of the movements.

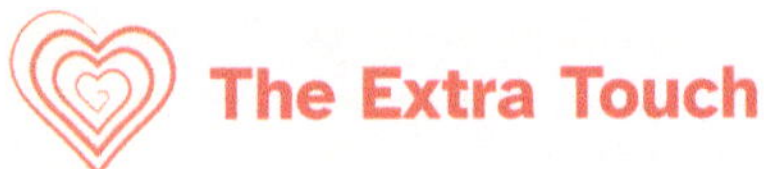

The Extra Touch

This position is very exciting for both partners. The man has a great view of his partner's entire body but cannot touch her. The woman, on the other hand, has complete freedom in her movements. She can lean forward or backward, caress all her erogenous zones as well as those of her partner.

The Supernova

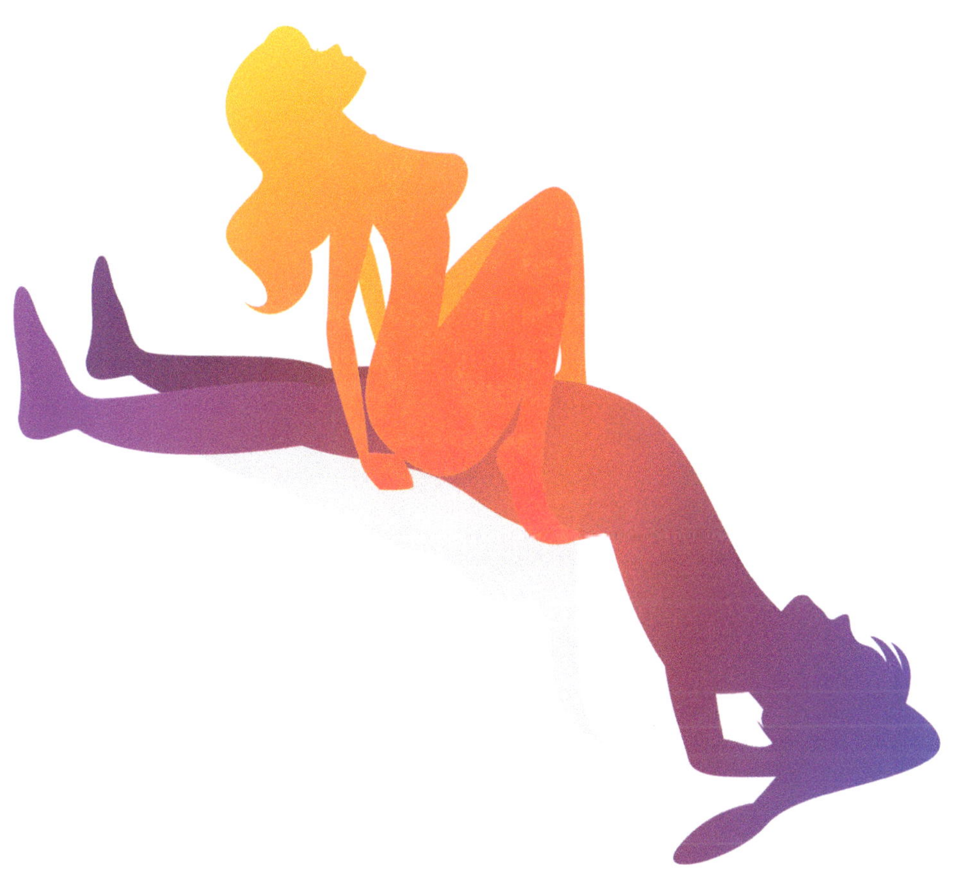

61

Suspended Congress:

The man stands, preferably against a wall, and lifts the woman. She wraps her arms around her lover's neck and squeezes her legs around his waist. During penetration, the man firmly holds onto the woman's buttocks and back and slightly bends his knees. The perfect position for a spontaneous encounter, with just the right amount of clothing removed, or for making love in a place other than home!

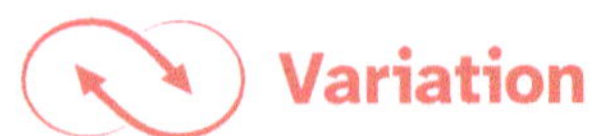 **Variation**

The couple adopts the same posture as the Stand-Up Lover, but the woman encircles her partner's waist with her legs for deeper penetration.

Suspended Congress

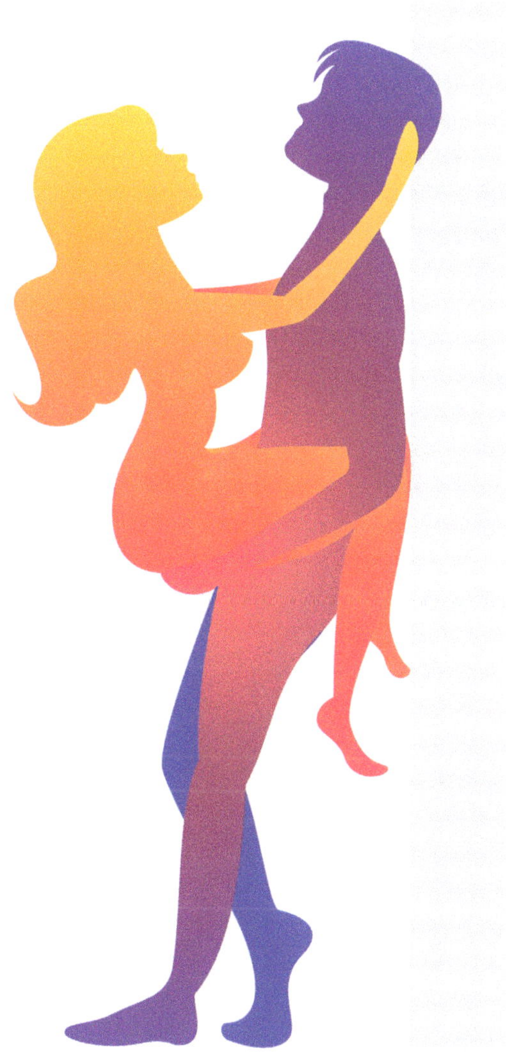

62

The G-Force:

The woman lies on her back, knees drawn towards her chest. The man, kneeling in front of her, takes hold of her feet and penetrates her by thrusting forward with his hips. To maintain her balance, the woman places her feet on her partner's chest and her hands on his thighs, while he holds her by the hips

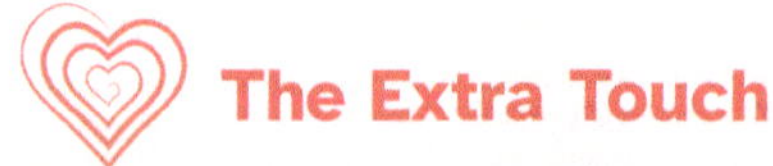 **The Extra Touch**

This position offers very deep and exciting penetration. For even more intensity, the man can caress the woman's breasts and clitoris.

The G-Force

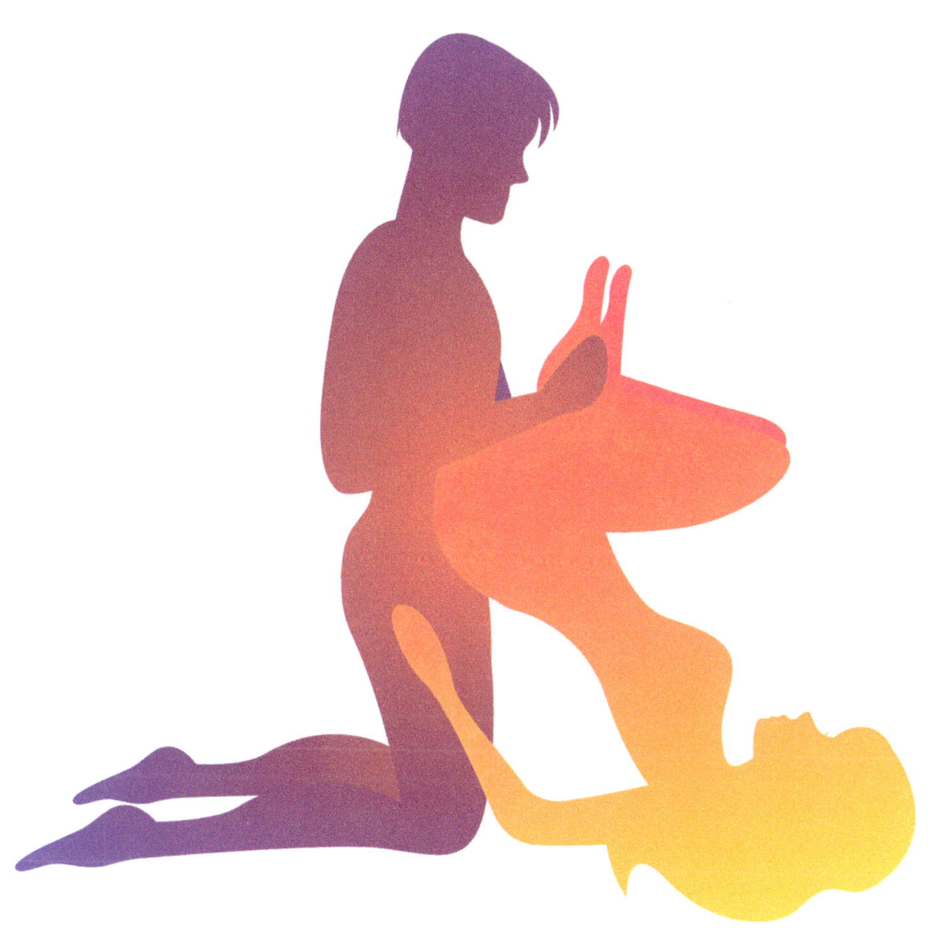

63

Folded Saint:

The woman lies on her back at the edge of the bed, legs spread, and feet on the floor. The man, kneeling, slips between her thighs. The woman then places her ankles on his shoulders while he lifts her torso. During penetration, the man firmly holds his partner in this position, placing one hand under her buttocks and the other on her back. The woman, in turn, wraps her arms around her lover's torso.

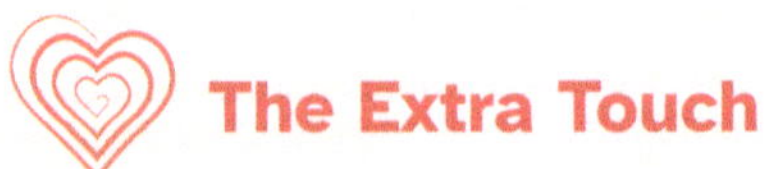 **The Extra Touch**

This position offers more than optimal depth of penetration but can quickly become tiring. The woman can be pressed against a wall for added comfort.

Folded Saint

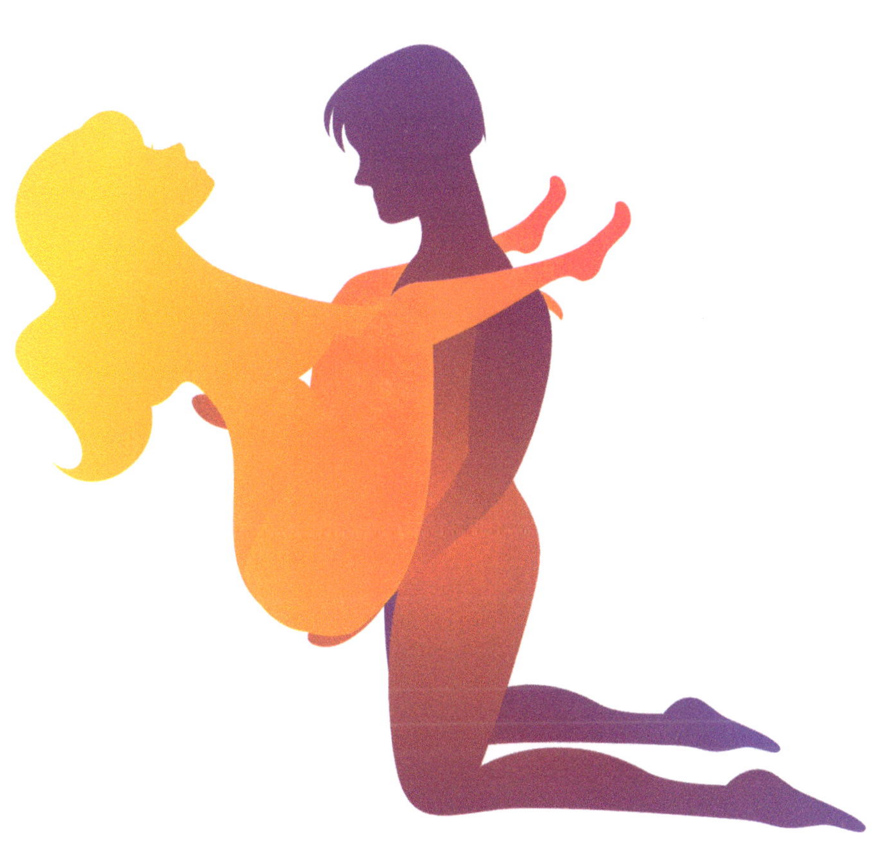

64

The Indian Handstand:

The woman bends forward, supporting herself on her hands with her arms extended. The man, standing behind her, lifts her pelvis while she slides her legs under his arms to hold onto him.

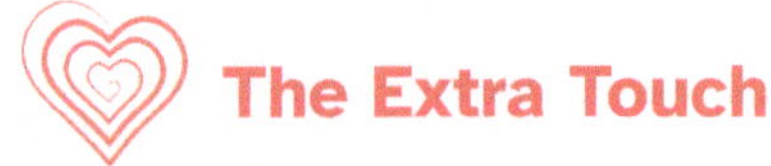 **The Extra Touch**

This position offers new sensations for both the man and the woman but requires strong arms. Perfect for getting some exercise while engaging in lovemaking!

The Indian Handstand

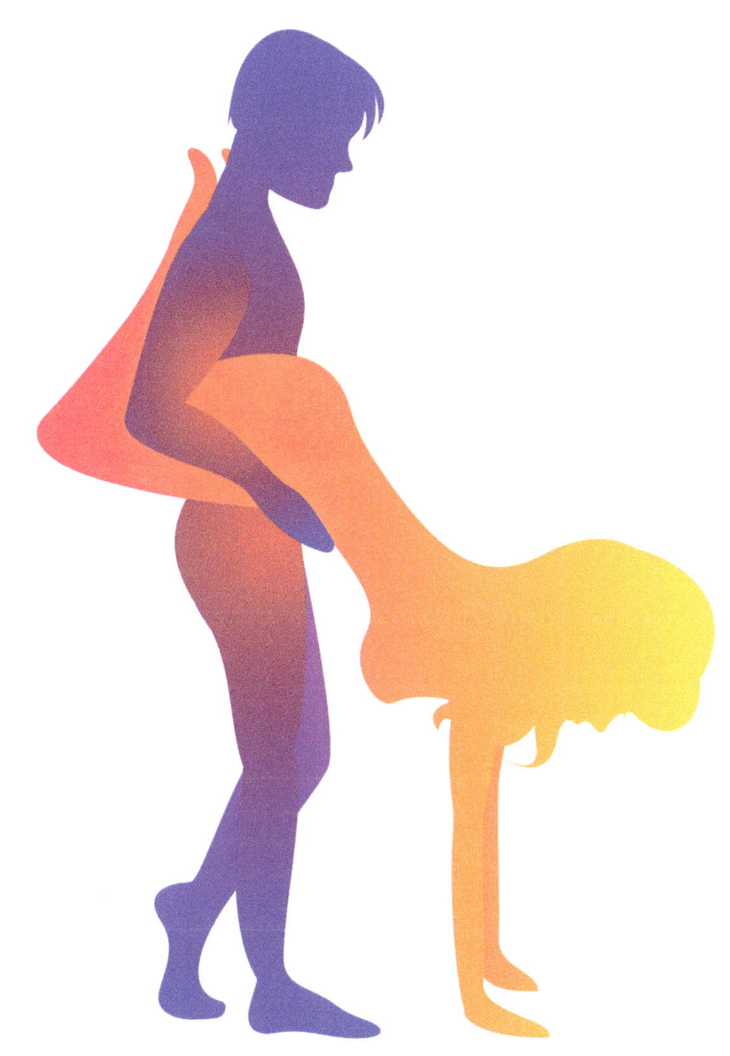

65

Balancing Act:

The man lies on his back with knees bent and legs spread. The woman sits on his lap, making sure not to crush him. The man holds her by the waist or buttocks to accompany her in a swinging motion, but she takes charge by setting the rhythm of the back-and-forth movements and controlling the depth of penetration.

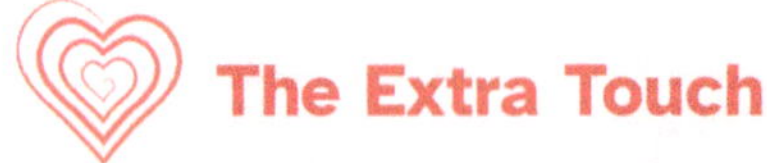

The Extra Touch

This position is very intense and requires perfect synchronization. The woman can also touch herself or stimulate her partner's perineum for even more pleasure.

Balancing Act

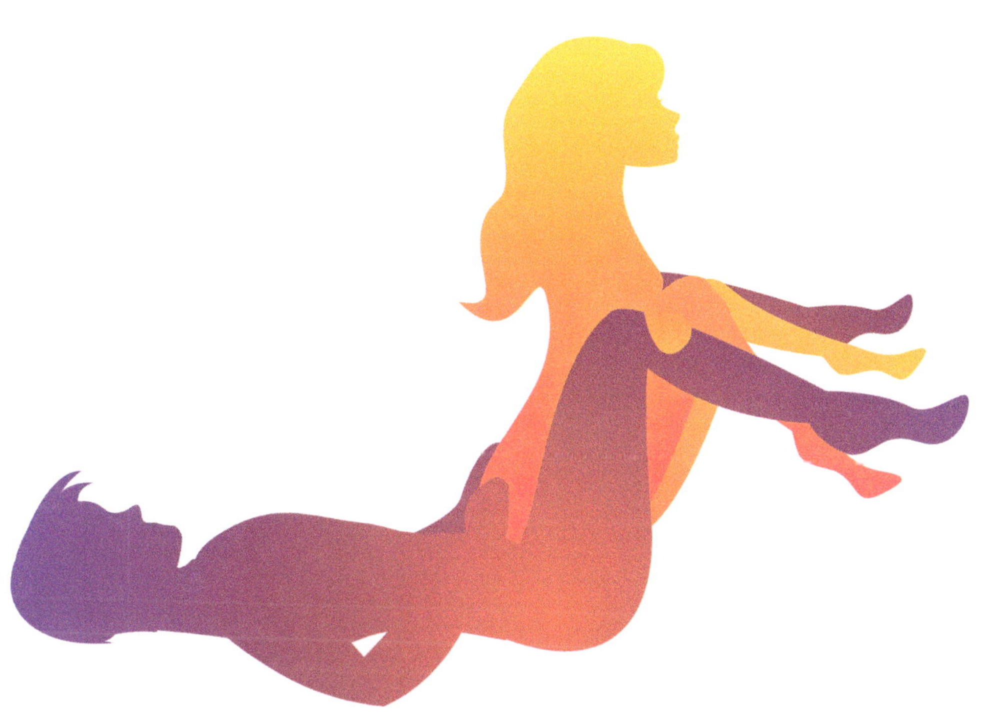

The Y Curve:

The woman lies face down on the edge of the bed, allowing her upper body to hang off the bed while her pelvis and legs rest on the bed. Her head and forearms are supported on the floor. The man lies on top of her, positioning himself between her legs. He then places his hands on her buttocks to lift her upper body and penetrates her.

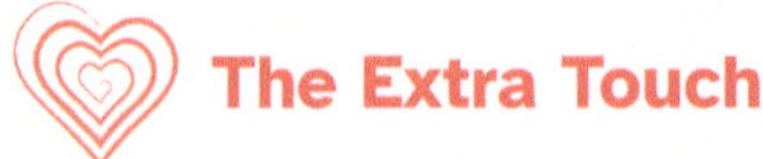

The Extra Touch

To enhance comfort, place a cushion under the woman's elbows.

The Y Curve

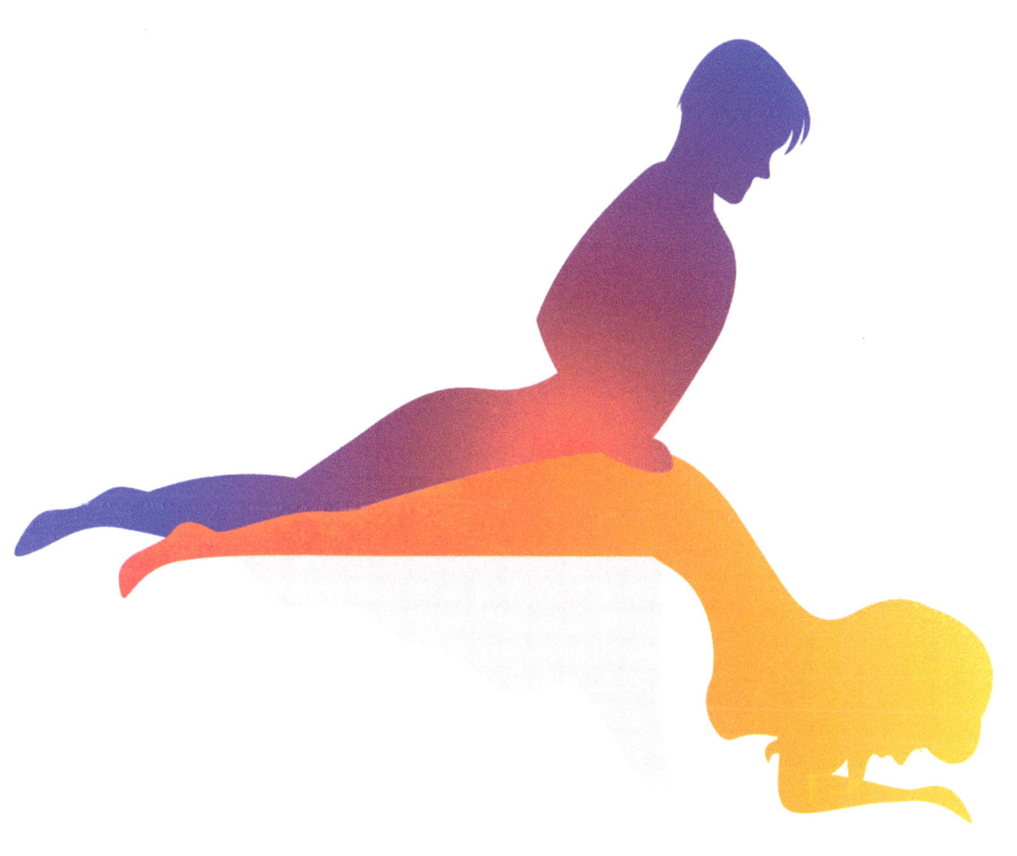

67

The pinwheel:

Both the man and the woman sit side by side so they can look at each other. The woman wraps her legs around the man's torso and relies on her hands to maintain balance. Her partner encircles her waist with his legs, holding her by the hips or thighs. They can then start with gentle up-and-down movements.

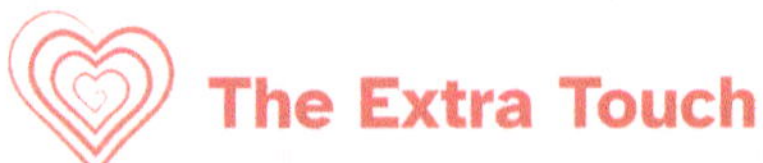

The Extra Touch

This position is more challenging than it appears, relying on the balance and support that both partners can provide to each other.

The pinwheel

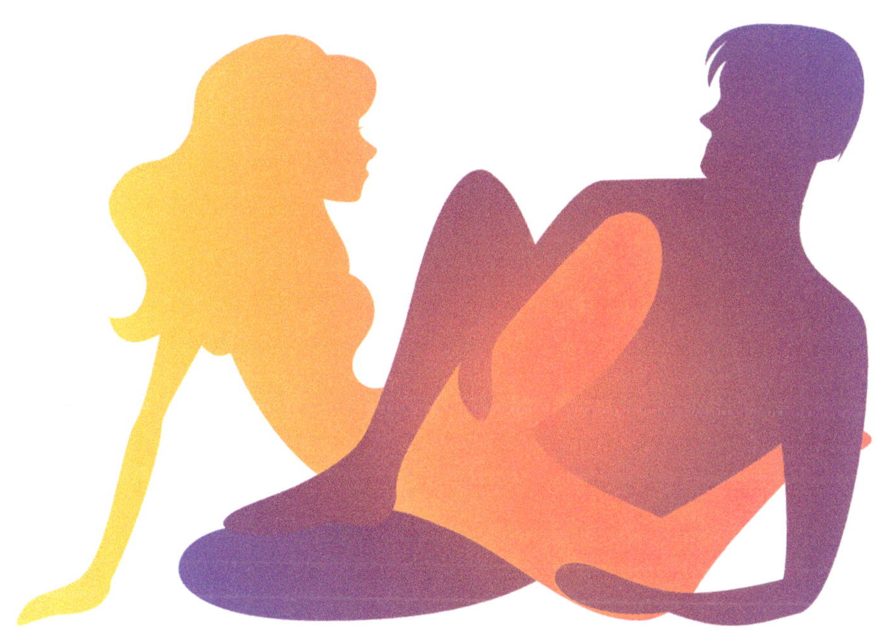

68

The Triuph Arc:

The man sits with his legs extended in front of him. The woman kneels facing him and then sits on his erect penis. After finding a comfortable position, arching her back, she lies down between her partner's legs. The man can then guide the movement of her hips and lean over to kiss her breasts and belly. With a free hand, he can caress other erogenous zones on her body.

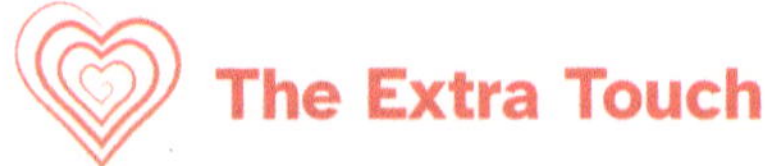 **The Extra Touch**

When excitement reaches its peak, the woman can raise her legs behind her partner to provide a stronger thrust during the back-and-forth motion.

The Triuph Arc

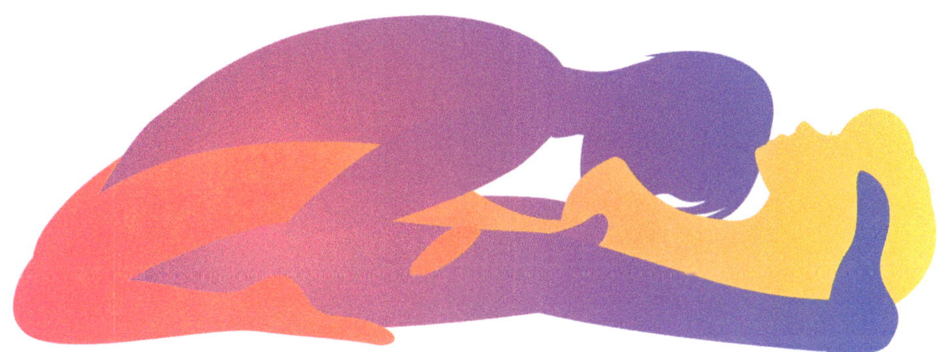

69

The Lustful Leg:

Both partners stand up. The woman grips the man's neck with her hands and raises one of her legs onto his shoulder. Her partner penetrates her while holding onto her buttocks.

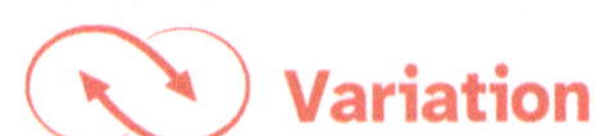 **Variation**

This position requires great flexibility. If the woman cannot place her leg on her partner's shoulder or if the position becomes tiring, she can lower her leg and wrap it around the man's hips.

The Lustful Leg

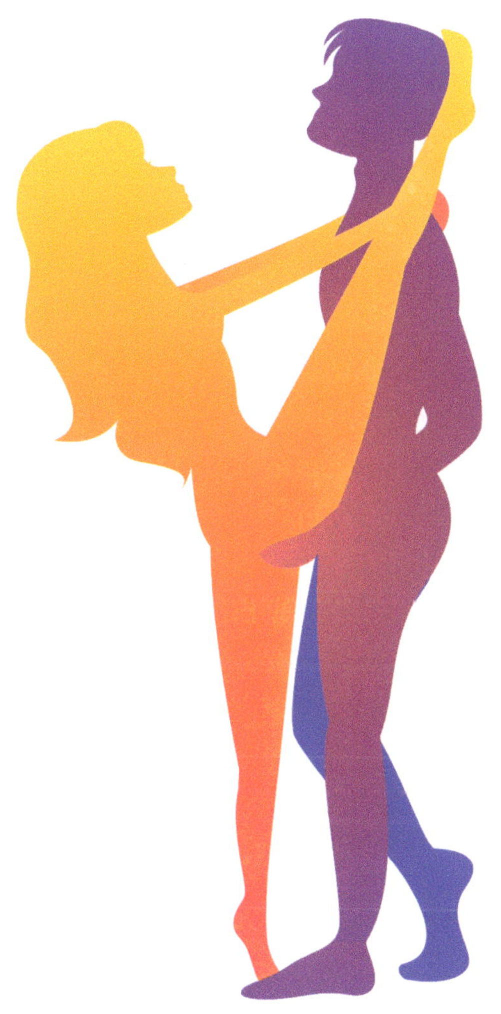

Conclusion

The End... or a New Beginning?

Congratulations, Love Adventurers! You've reached the end of "The Sex Positions Challenge." But remember, "Your Sex Positions Challenge" is not just a game to finish. It's a journey to revisit, over and over again. Your scores can always be improved, new variations or practices can be invented, and new locations can be explored. By breaking the routine, you'll bring a spark back into your relationship. So step out of your comfort zone; the adventure is just beginning!

Laugh, love, experiment, and, most importantly, keep rising to "Your Sex Positions Challenge," over and over again!

Stay tuned for new naughty adventures!